CLINICAL PROBLEMS IN PEDIATRIC AND ADOLESCENT GYNECOLOGY

Provided as an educational service by

Wyeth-Ayerst Laboratories

World Leadership in
Women's Health Care ®

**WYETH-AYERST
LABORATORIES**
Philadelphia, PA 19101

CLINICAL PROBLEMS IN PEDIATRIC AND ADOLESCENT GYNECOLOGY

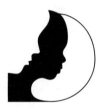

Edited by
Alvin F. Goldfarb, M.D.
Professor of Obstetrics and Gynecology
Director, Medical Education Department of Obstetrics and Gynecology
Jefferson Medical College of Thomas Jefferson University
Philadelphia, Pennsylvania

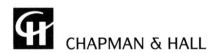
CHAPMAN & HALL

An International Thomson Publishing Company
New York • Albany • Bonn • Boston • Cincinnati • Detroit • London • Madrid • Melbourne
Mexico City • Pacific Grove • Paris • San Francisco • Singapore • Tokyo • Toronto • Washington

Cover Design: Andrea Meyer, emDASH Inc.

Copyright © 1996 by Chapman & Hall, New York, NY

Printed in the United States of America

For more information contact:

Chapman & Hall
115 Fifth Avenue
New York, NY 10003

Chapman & Hall
2-6 Boundary Row
London SE1 8HN
England

Thomas Nelson Australia
102 Dodds Street
South Melbourne, 3205
Victoria, Australia

Chapman & Hall GmbH
Postfach 100 263
D-69442 Weinheim
Germany

International Thomson Editores
Campos Eliseos 385, Piso 7
Col. Polanco
11560 Mexico D.F.
Mexico

International Thomson Publishing - Japan
Hirakawacho-cho Kyowa Building, 3F
1-2-1 Hirakawacho-cho
Chiyoda-ku, 102 Tokyo
Japan

International Thomson Publishing Asia
221 Henderson Road #05-10
Henderson Building
Singapore 0315

2 3 4 5 6 7 8 9 XXX 01 00 99 98 97

Library of Congress Cataloging-in-Publication Data
Clinical probelms in pediatric and adolescent gynecology / [edited by] Alvin F. Goldfarb.
           p.   cm.
  Includes bibliographical references and index.
  ISBN 0-412-07201-7 (alk. paper)
  1. Pediatric gynecology. 2. Adolescent gynecology. I. Goldfarb, Alvin F. (Alvin Frank), 1923--
  [DNLM: 1. Genital Diseases, Female--in infancy & childhood. 2. Genital Diseases, Female--in adolescence. 3. Genitalia, Female.
  4. Child Abuse, Sexual. 5. Physical Examination. 6. Puberty--physiology. 7. Sex Behavior--in adolescence. WS 360 C641 1996]
  RJ478.C55   1996
  618.92'098--dc20
  DNLM/DLC   96-13866
  for Library of Congress   CIP

Visit Chapman & Hall on the Internet http://www.chaphall.com/chaphall.html

To order this or any other Chapman & Hall book, please contact **International Thomson Publishing, 7625 Empire Drive, Florence, KY 41042.** Phone (606) 525-6600 or 1-800-842-3636. Fax: (606) 525-7778. E-mail: order@chaphall.com.

For a complete listing of Chapman & Hall titles, send your request to **Chapman & Hall, Dept. BC, 115 Fifth Avenue, New York, NY 10003.**

To all the millions of young girls who require gynecologic care—and their health care providers.

North American Society for Pediatric
and Adolescent Gynecology

CONTENTS

PREFACE

In 1967, I participated in a New York Academy of Science program devoted to pediatric and adolescent gynecology. The chairman of the program was my late good friend Warren R. Lang, M.D. Approximately 50 years ago, Warren and I ran the colposcopy clinic at the Jefferson Medical College Hospital Out-Patient Service. In his introduction to the annals covering this meeting on pediatric and adolescent gynecology, Warren wrote the following, "This volume represents the first major attempt to review attitudes, research and progress in the field of pediatric and adolescent gynecology. Only recently has a general interest in gynecology of the pediatric patient become evident despite the classic textbook by Schauffler now in its fourth edition. At present, most textbooks on gynecology may have merely mentioned the area of pediatric and adolescent gynecology." Have we made any progress in three decades? How many meaningful textbooks have evolved in this period of time concerning this subject? How many medical schools have even curriculum concerning this subject? How may clinics are there in the country that talk about this subject and manage patients with these problems? How many fellowships are there in the country that deal with the problems of pediatric and adolescent gynecology? These questions still have not received positive answers. It is the purpose of this book to provide information that will allow the health care provider to answer these questions and improve care for these patients.

This book—which is divided into three sections—presents in the first section the management of clinical problems related to vulvo-vaginal disease and sexual abuse. The second section deals with the physiology of puberty and the management of abnormal uterine bleeding. The third portion of the book reviews for the reader the problems that deal with adolescent sexuality and managing human papilloma virus (HPV). As a final chapter an excellent review of the differential diagnosis and management of pelvic pain. The reader should be aware of the fact that no attempt was made to write these chapters in a monolithic fashion. Therefore each chapter is written in the style of the author and each has its own flavor. I would hope, therefore, that the reader will not get bored with this book.

The first portion of this book deals with the patient and the examination and problems that relate to the vulvo-vaginal area of her body. In the very first chapter Dr. Yordan points out with clarity, based upon experience, the tips and tricks that can be used to examine any pediatric and adolescent gynecologic patient. Among the most important points made in this article is one should never embarrass or hurt the patient, but rather empower the patient to participate in the examination, always keeping in mind that the examination should be part of an educational process. There is much wonderful material in this particular chapter. Following this chapter, Dr. Janice Bacon introduces us to the subject of vulvo-vaginitis.

This chapter is quite clear, allows for us to understand the biology of the vagina, the development of the vulvo-vaginal area, and reviews in depth the differential diagnosis of clinical problems. With a proper diagnosis, the management of the disease becomes quite easy. It is during these first two chapters that one begins to understand the intricacies of pediatric and adolescent gynecology. Unfortunately, these patients have never had a clinic area developed for them. Most of our attitudes relate to the development of clinics with the adult in mind rather than the pediatric and adolescent gynecologic patient.

Among the pioneers working with children who are exposed to sexual assault was Dr. Vincent Capraro. He defined for us the procedures for the work-up of the sexually assaulted female. Since Capraro's work in the early 60's there has been a growth in our understanding of sexual abuse and sexual assault in the pediatric and adolescent patient. Dr. Susan Pokorny, presently President of NASPAG, in her unusually clear manner reviewed pediatric sexual abuse. The development of evidence, understanding the balancing of the history and physical findings and conducting an evidentiary medical examination are concisely reported. The emotional travail that the child goes through in the management of the problem is discussed with empathy and understanding by the writer. The development of a comfort index among health care providers to understand the trauma that is associated with sexual abuse and the ability to have balance in deciding whether or not sexual abuse has occurred is well documented. This balance must be understood by all individuals who see patients with this problem.

The next two chapters deal with normal pubescence and one of the more common problems seen in the adolescent gynecologic patient, excess uterine bleeding. Peter Lee has done a masterful job in defining the normal endocrine mechanisms that are associated with pubescence and the development of the normal menstrual cycle. The information in this chapter is well written, up to date, and reads easily. Included in his review of pubertal development and the physiology of the hypothalamic pituitary gonadal axis is new information regarding growth factors and their relationship to menstrual function. The tables and the graphs certainly make the chapter enjoyable reading.

Your editor had the easiest part in the development of this book and that was to write a chapter on abnormal uterine bleeding. The important points to remember in this chapter are that bleeding which the individual presents with is only a symptom, and it is our responsibility with a proper history and physical examination to define the etiology of the bleeding. The management of this problem is presented in algorithm form which allows the clinician to work through the management of any patient who presents with abnormal uterine bleeding.

The last part of the book deals with problems of adolescent sexuality. These chapters include the development of adolescent sexuality, as written by Dr. Brown. In addition there are chapters on the role of contraception and of sexually transmitted diseases that may have serious consequences as a precursor to the development of carcinoma of the cervix-HPV. As Dr. Brown points out, the development of sexuality during adolescence is the summation of environmental and biological factors and social factors, including family relationship and attitudes as well as cultural and societal norms and expectations. If the process proceeds well the young person will achieve adulthood with a good sense of self—as a woman or as a man—in the capacity to form meaningful and lasting relationships. This chapter is well written and presents information in a simple succinct manner.

And lastly, the story of Human Papilloma Virus and its implication and its effect on adolescents is reviewed. The important portion of this chapter is that the clinician should not take the Papanicolaou report as dogma, but should place it in perspective with the physical findings. Repeating the smear might be a worthwhile step before moving ahead and involving the patient in all forms of therapeutic procedures which may not be necessary.

To compliment this chapter on HPV, what about the other STD's? The other STD's really were not reviewed, but instead we thought it would be nice to balance off the book with a chapter on pelvic pain, both acute and chronic. Dr. Kozlowski has done an excellent job in putting this in perspective and including a review of pelvic inflammatory disease.

If one were to compare the annals of the New York Academy of Science, Volume 142, pages 547–834 on pediatric and adolescent gynecology as published in 1967 and this current book, we can see that we have gone from the endocrine and organic with minimal behavioral concerns regarding the patient to a balance involving an understanding of the endocrine and organic causes of the disease, but modified in treatment with a behavioral attitude.

The purpose of this book is to share with you, the reader, as much information as possible so that your decision making processes in managing some of the clinical problems seen in the area of pediatric and adolescent gynecology will be improved. We trust that the information will serve you in such a fashion that there will be an improved partnership that will develop between the patient, her family and you—thus leading to improved care for the pediatric and adolescent gynecologic patient.

Alvin F. Goldfarb, M.D.

CONTRIBUTORS

James Bacon, M.D.
USC Richland Memorial Hospital
2 Richland Med. Park, Suite 302
Columbia, SC 29203

Robert Brown, M.D.
Ohio State College of Medicine
Section for Adolescent Health
700 Children's Drive
Columbus, OH 43205

Janice L. Goerzen, M.D.
University of Calgary
Foothills Hospital, Department
   Obstetrics/Gynecology
1403 29th Street, NW
Calgary, Alberta
Canada T2N 2T9

Alvin F. Goldfarb, M.D.
Department of Obstetrics/Gynecology
Jefferson Medical College of Thomas
   Jefferson University
Philadelphia, PA 19107

Karen J. Kozlowski, M.D.
4501 Lile Drive, Suite 770
Little Rock, Arkansas 72205

Peter Lee, M.D.
Children's Hospital of Pittsburgh
3705 Fifth Avenue
Pittsburgh, PA 15213–2583

Susan F. Pokorny, M.D.
Department of Obstetrics/Gynecology
Baylor College of Medicine
One Baylor Plaza
Houston, TX 77030

Walter D. Rosenfeld, M.D.
Adolescent Service
Morristown Memorial Hosp
100 Madison Ave
Morristown, NJ 07962

Elaine Yordan, M.D.
St. Francis Hospital and Medical Center
Department of Pediatrics, Society of
   Adolescent Medicine
114 Woodland Street
Hartford, Connecticut 06105

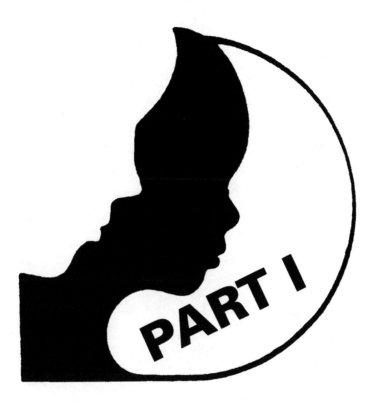

TIPS, TRICKS, AND TESTS FOR THE GYNECOLOGIC EXAM OF YOUNG FEMALES

Elaine E. Yordan, M.D.

INTRODUCTION

A comprehensive knowledge of pediatric genital and anal anatomy is essential for practitioners of pediatric and adolescent gynecology. To increase the likelihood that the gynecologic examination will provide thorough, accurate information, practitioners also must master strategies that enhance the comfort and cooperation of their patients. In this chapter, I share some of the techniques and routines that I employ and find valuable in the gynecologic examination of young female patients.

The approach that I take to the patient is very much dependent on her age and level of development. Even though there is some overlap, I find it helpful to think of patients as falling into one of three age categories: preschool and elementary school, middle school, and adolescence.

THE GENERAL SETTING

The general setting for the examination is very important. Not surprisingly, the chaos and confusion of the emergency room make it a suboptimal location. The appropriate atmosphere in the waiting area should be calming and unhurried. In the same manner that a surgeon allows extra time for a complex operative case, you should set aside ample time in your office schedule when seeing pediatric gynecology patients. Extraneous distractions can be detrimental. You need to be focused and concentrating, as the findings have both medical and potential legal importance.

THE PRESCHOOL/ELEMENTARY SCHOOL AGE PATIENT

There are a variety of reasons why girls in preschool and elementary school are referred for a gynecologic examination. These commonly include dermatologic conditions of the vulva, vaginal discharge, itching and scratching, suspected blood on panties, vulvar dysuria, and alleged sexual abuse.

Initial Contact with the Parent

Members of your office staff must be trained to interact successfully over the telephone with the parent (usually the mother) who calls to make the appointment. Staff should describe the examination and use of colposcope, emphasizing that the instrument is not inserted into the patient. The parent must be reassured that the examination is not painful. It is important for the mother to understand how a pediatric gynecologic examination differs from that to which she is accustomed. The mother also should be advised about how to prepare her daughter for the upcoming appointment. Of course, the explanation given to the child depends on her age.

A simple and accurate approach is best: "Today, we are going to see the doctor. She will look at the outside of your vagina to find out why you have been itching so much." The mother should explain to the child that the examination will not hurt and that there will be no injections. It is also helpful for the child to bring a favorite doll or stuffed animal along for comfort and security. I recommend that a trusted adult relative or friend accompany the mother and child as a source of support.

When the chief complaint is a vaginal discharge in this age group, I suggest to the mother that the child not be bathed for 24 hours before the examination. If there are any findings on the child's panties, the panties should be presented at the time of the appointment for inspection.

Interviewing the Mother

For this age group, I find it ideal to interview the mother alone to take a medical/social history and discuss the examination (Figure 1-1). Your office is probably not "child-proof" and it can be particularly distracting if the child is exuberantly romping about. Interviewing the mother alone is especially important in cases of alleged sexual abuse because subjective statements that the mother makes in the presence of the child may influence how the child recounts details of the abuse. In addition, if you speak to the parents in the presence of the child, they may not be readily forthcoming about sensitive family issues that could have an important bearing on the case.

A private conversation is possible only if the child will separate from the mother without difficulty. If separation provokes a tearful reaction from the child, a private talk with the mother may not be possible. Many parents believe that their child will not separate easily, but surprisingly most children are quite happy to accompany a nurse to a play area. It is not unusual for the child to periodically return to peek into your consultation room just to make sure that Mom is still there. The time the child spends in the play area also provides an excellent opportunity for your nurse to assess the child's developmental level and to determine how best to relate to her (Figure 1-2). Occasionally, a mother may object to her child being alone in the play area with

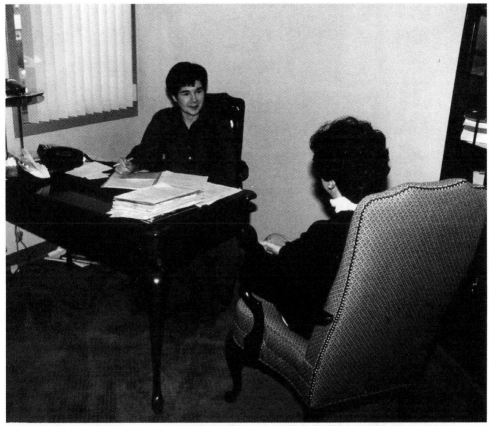

Figure 1-1. It is important to interview the young patient's mother alone, explain the scope of the examination, and provide assurances of your support and understanding.

your nurse who is a stranger to her. In these circumstances it is useful for a relative or trusted friend to stay with the child in the waiting room.

Before you bring the mother and daughter into the examination room, it is important that the mother understand how her daughter's exam will differ from the gynecologic examination of an adult. If the mother is anxious and tearful, the child will react similarly. This can happen if the mother herself has a history of sexual abuse or sexual assault and remembers her own examination as having been negative or traumatic. Sometimes, what may appear to be a simple complaint of a vaginal discharge may in fact be a highly volatile subject. The vaginal discharge may have become the overriding concern at home. The parents may have become obsessed with the problem and you may be the third or fourth physician they have consulted. In these instances, they will need your support and understanding to deal with the emotional feelings that the situation has provoked.

Establishing Rapport with the Patient

After speaking with the mother, I have her accompany me back to the waiting room and extend my hand to the little girl inviting her to return with us to my office (Figure

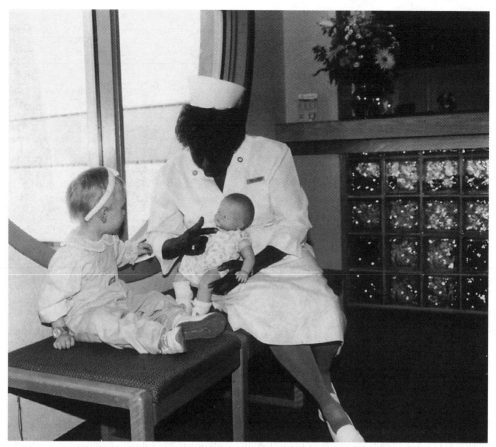

Figure 1-2.   An experienced nurse can be extremely helpful in assessing the patient's developmental level and how best to relate to her.

1-3). In these situations I do not wear my customary white lab coat. Depending on the patient's intellectual and developmental level, it may or may not be possible to take a history from her. You can talk about whatever might interest her: the doll she brought with her, a familiar television character, or perhaps the outfit she is wearing.

This time provides an excellent opportunity to establish some physical contact with the patient (Figure 1-4). I will usually attempt to gently touch her hand during the conversation. I watch the child's body language carefully and relate to her accordingly.

When speaking with the mother, I believe it is important to use correct terminology for the genitalia, making careful distinction between the vulva and vagina. However, when interacting with the child I prefer to use her terminology and usually ask the mother which words the child uses to refer to the vulva and perianal area. I then can discuss the reason for the examination using the child's vocabulary. For example, "I need to take a look at your pee-pee because Mommy tells me you have itching down there. Why don't you, Mommy, and your little doll come over here to this special table?"

No matter what the indication for the examination, my approach to the patient

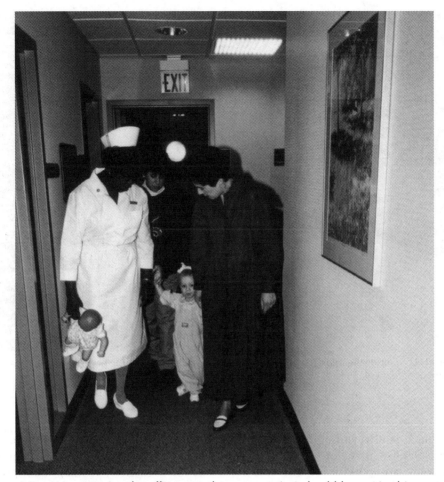

Figure 1-3. Upon entering the office area, the young patient should be received in a warm and supportive manner.

remains the same. However, it is important to keep in mind that there may be significant psychological factors affecting a child who has been sexually or physically abused.

I usually ask the mother to remain in the room during the examination. One exception is the rare occasion when the mother has said that the child will behave better if she is not present. Another exception is a case of reported sexual abuse in which the mother is the alleged perpetrator. In this instance the child may be accompanied by another supportive person such as a rape crisis counselor, a child protective services social worker, or perhaps the child's therapist.

If you plan to photograph or videotape for documentation, it is important to know if a sexual abuse case, for example, involved pornography. Even if you have consent from the parent, in cases involving child pornography you have to be certain that the child is comfortable being photographed. I find that children age 5 and older can understand the explanation of the medical and legal purposes of photo documentation.

The mother should help the child to get undressed and put on the examination gown.

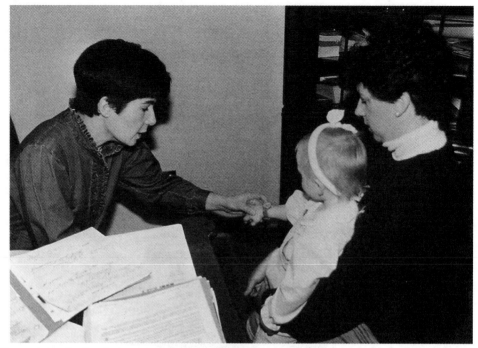

Figure 1-4. During the interview it is important to gently establish some preliminary physical contact with the young patient.

I find that it is always helpful to have a pediatric examination gown with a cheerful pattern such as clowns or teddy bears available for the patient. Respect for autonomy and privacy is important for little kids, too, and it is necessary to keep them properly draped. The child doesn't need to be completely undressed, and she usually can keep a T-shirt and socks on. Explain to the child what you will be doing. Depending on the situation, it is a good idea to examine her doll first. When the patient is ready, I generally first lift up the T-shirt and listen to her heart and lungs, and then palpate her breast, abdomen, and inguinal regions. This part of the examination further establishes physical contact with the patient. I deliberately avoid examination of the ears or throat as patients may react negatively if they find this uncomfortable.

Preparing for the Examination

Just as the nurse in the operating room plays a critical role, my nurse knows how to anticipate exactly what I will need. She is very much like the nurse in the operating room efficiently snapping instruments into the surgeon's hands. Most importantly, the nurse, whose name should be recorded in the medical record, is a witness to what occurs during the examination.

During most of this time the nurse and I are quietly singing songs familiar to preschool children. The commercially available combination teddy bear and cassette tape player

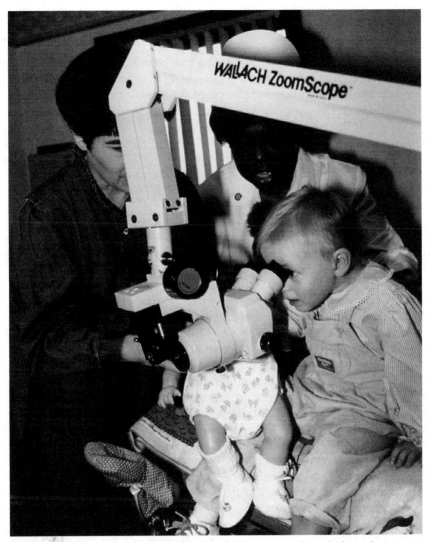

Figure 1-5. It is important to allow the child to see and touch the colposcope.

called "Mr. Spinoza" is a particular favorite of my patients.* In addition to playing songs, this device can be hugged and can be used to demonstrate the knee chest position. We try to relax the child by talking about her favorite activities, foods, and holidays. We encourage her to sing a favorite song and sing along with her.

The colposcope is always a helpful tool for this examination as a source of light and magnification. All gynecologists usually have one handy. It is noninvasive and painless. It is important to allow the child to see and touch the colposcope (Figure 1-5). You

---

*Spinoza™, 245 East 6th Street, St. Paul, MN 55101-1940. 1-800-282-2327.

can shine the colposcope light on her fingers. She can look at her doll through the colposcope. I flash the colposcope light across the walls of the room, and we pretend that it is Tinker Bell from Peter Pan.

I personally have difficulty accomplishing a good examination with the child on the mother's lap and find that this position is good only for a brief look at the vulva. There may be no alternative, however, for the child who resists being on the examination table. Nevertheless, in my opinion, the child needs to be in a position that facilitates visual inspection. If the patient is still in diapers, the frog-leg position is good, particularly because she is already accustomed to it. As the mother removes her diaper the child naturally assumes this position. Otherwise, I find it convenient to examine the patient in stirrups with the mother at the side of the examination table by the child's head.

Examining the Patient

The nurse and I tell the patient that the nurse will be touching the outside of her genitalia to help me see. In this respect the nurse's hands will be my hands. I believe that this technique plays a key role in the success of my examination technique. During the gynecologic examination I *never* actually touch the patient. My nurse begins by providing gentle lateral labial separation and proceeds to provide traction while I inspect the tissue through the colposcope. The vestibule, hymen, and lower third of the vagina are easily visualized by placing separation then traction on the labia majora.

If cultures are to be taken, I place my hand against the nurse's hand for support (Figure 1-6). This avoids any additional and potentially disquieting tactile stimulus to the patient. To obtain a culture specimen, I use a sterile nasopharyngeal calcium alginate tipped applicator moistened with sterile nonbacteriostatic normal saline. I pass the applicator into the vagina without touching the rim of the hymen (Figure 1-7). Any specimen to be tested for the presence of *Neiserria gonorrhoeae* and *Chlamydia trachomatis* should be placed, respectively, on Thayer Martin medium and McCoy Cell medium.[1,2] To obtain a throat culture for *Neiserria gonorrhoeae* from young children, I compare the culture swab to a toothbrush and tell them that I will begin by touching their back molar. After positioning the swab on the back molar, I then pass the swab medially to the posterior tonsillar pillar and then onto the posterior pharyngeal wall.

The degree to which I examine the patient is dependent upon the situation. For example, if the symptom of itching or scratching is found to be the result of lichen sclerosis and the hymen appears normal, then no cultures are necessary. It is also important to take a careful look at the anus. If the chief complaint includes a vaginal discharge, possible foreign body, possible bleeding, or alleged sexual abuse, it is also necessary to examine the patient in the knee chest position. In this instance, again, it is very important that the nurse be skilled in eliciting the maximal voluntary cooperation from the patient. Proper positioning of the patient by the nurse will maximize your opportunity for visual inspection with the colposcope. In the knee-chest position the child's shoulders should be down on the examining table, with her head turned toward the mother, buttocks in the air, with the back swayed, and knees spread apart enough so that the umbilicus is visible to the examiner (Figure 1-8). The knee-chest position is familiar to toddlers and very young children as they commonly sleep in this position; the mother in the examination room may remind the child of this.

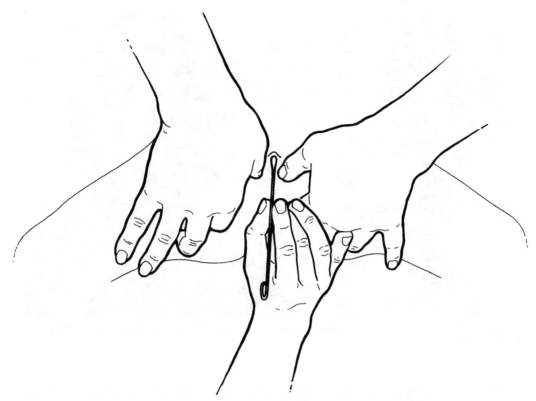

Figure 1-6. Technique by which the author supports her hand against the nurse's hand during the acquisition of specimens from the prepubertal vagina. (Shown without examining gloves for purposes of illustration.)

Evaluation of Vaginal Discharges

It is important to ask the mother to bring the patient's panties to the examination if any discharge has been reported, especially blood. To determine if there is blood in a discharge, moisten the stained area of the panties with normal saline, rub this on a stool guaiac card, and test the sample for blood according to the manufacturer's instructions. I have found red stains on panties to be ketchup, cosmetics, and magic marker.

Removal of Foreign Objects from the Vagina

A foreign object in the vagina can be the cause of vaginal discharge in young girls. A simple procedure for removing a foreign object involves irrigation of warmed sterile normal saline flushed into the vagina through a 50-cc syringe attached to a small-caliber infant feeding tube. Tactile stimulus of the patient is minimized by passing the tip of the infant feeding tube through the hymenal orifice into the vagina without touching the rim of the hymen. While the feeding tube is held in place, firm pressure is applied to the syringe; the foreign material usually is passed as the irrigation fluid escapes from the vagina. Any recovered material should be sent for pathological examination. It is

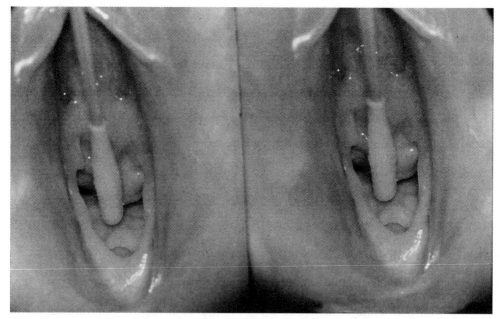

Figure 1-7.   A calcium alginate–tipped applicator passing into the vagina without touching the rim of the hymen.

important for the examiner to be wearing a face mask and goggles because of the risk of being splashed during this procedure.

Collection of Vaginal Secretions

Secretions from the prepubertal vagina can be collected in several ways. If a secretion is pooled in the vagina, you can use a sterile disposable plastic dropper to dilute it with sterile nonbacteriostatic normal saline and then aspirate the fluid. Another technique for removing secretions from the prepubertal vagina uses irrigation and an easy-to-construct double-lumen catheter.[3] Any vaginal discharge should be tested for *Neiserria gonorrhoeae, Chlamydia trachomatis,* and other bacterial growth. If an adequate specimen is obtained a wet preparation should be performed.

Sedation and Anesthesia

On rare occasions, sedation or anesthesia may be necessary during the gynecologic examination. Procedural sedation with Midazolam for preschool and elementary school age patients has been described.[4] Local anesthesia can be used in conjunction with the evaluation and treatment of superficial vulvar and perineal lacerations. Viscous lidocaine (2%) can be gently applied to such a wound with excellent results. General anesthesia is necessary when a vaginal bleeding source cannot be otherwise identified and/or controlled, when a known foreign body cannot otherwise be removed, and when it is necessary to evaluate penetrating trauma to the vagina.

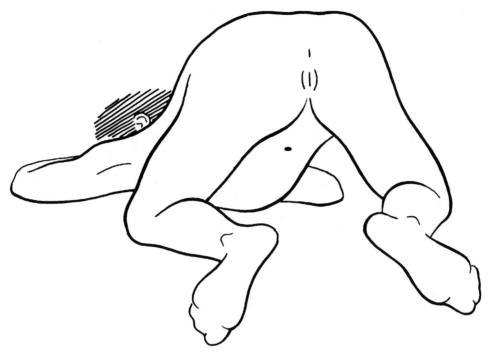

Figure 1-8. Optimal posture for the knee-chest position. Note that the child's shoulders are down on the examining table, with her head turned toward the mother, buttocks in the air, back swayed, and knees spread apart enough so that the umbilicus is visible to the examiner.

THE MIDDLE SCHOOL AGE PATIENT

Patients in the middle school group usually are 10 to 12 years of age. They may have Tanner 3 or 4 breasts and may not have reached menarche. I find that these patients are particularly shy and modest, as they tend to be uncomfortable with the changes taking place in the appearance of their bodies. In my experience, common indications for a gynecologic examination in this age group include discharge (usually a physiologic leukorrhea), vulvitis, concern about the appearance of the breasts, concern about the appearance of the external genitalia, concern that menarche has not taken place, vaginal bleeding (usually menarche), trauma, and alleged sexual abuse.

Establishing Rapport with the Patient

For these patients, history taking will obviously be different than with preschoolers. Because you are not the patient's regular health care provider and do not have an established relationship with her, it is important to develop a comfortable, sympathetic, trustworthy environment for both the patient and her mother. It is appropriate to take the chief complaint and the history from the Mother, but it is necessary to include the girl in this process as well. How you do this depends upon the circumstances and how the girl is reacting to them. In many cases of alleged sexual abuse in this age group, the patient may not want to repeat, yet again, the story that brings her to you. This is not a problem if she previously has been interviewed by child protective services or the police. All you really need to do is focus on her general health and the examination.

Interviewing the Patient

Speaking to the girl alone is valuable because she may want to tell you something that she hasn't told her mother. For example, when sexual abuse is not suspected, the girl may reveal a history of sexual abuse for the first time to you or tell you that the perpetrator is still in the home. In cases not involving sexual abuse, the mother may not know all her daughter's worries and concerns. For example, the girl may reveal to you that she is voluntarily sexually active.

If the patient is worried about pregnancy or sexually transmitted diseases, you will need to discuss these subjects. I have seen a number of premenarchal girls truly worried about having become pregnant after being sexually abused in ways that would not result in a pregnancy. In addition to explaining how the abuse could not result in a pregnancy, it is very appropriate to immediately perform a urine pregnancy test with the patient watching and show her the negative result.

Speaking to the mother alone at some point also is useful. For example, in a case of alleged sexual abuse, the mother may want to talk privately about some sensitive issues in her own life, such as a personal history of abuse.

Preparing for the Examination

As for the examination itself, the girl may or may not want the mother to be present, so I leave that decision to her. It is important to discuss the nature of the examination not only with the mother but also with the girl. It is very helpful to use pictures, models, and diagrams of pelvic anatomy as part of the discussion. In cases of alleged sexual abuse, I like to have my nurse present as my assistant and chaperone.

Because, as noted, patients in this age group tend to be shy and modest, I am always careful to respect those feelings in the examination room. During the general part of the examination, the appropriate use of gowns and drapes should be observed. Here too, pleasant conversation may help to relax the patient.

Examinating the Patient

If the girl is not sexually active, a speculum examination is usually not necessary. If the girl is voluntarily sexually active or the chief complaint involves alleged sexual abuse by penile vaginal penetration, then a speculum examination should be done. Remember, this will be the patient's first gynecologic examination and, I believe, may have a lasting influence on her attitude toward gynecologic health care. So the exam should be as gentle as possible. Assure the girl that if she has discomfort during the exam, you will stop immediately.

You should use a Huffman speculum or a Pederson speculum (Figure 1-9).[5] A preg-

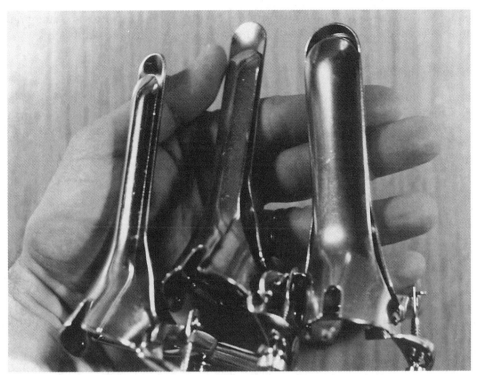

Figure 1-9. From left to right: a Huffman vaginal speculum, a Pederson vaginal speculum, and a Graves vaginal speculum.

nancy test should be done if there is any possibility of pregnancy. If a speculum examination is performed, a Pap smear should be obtained. For medico-legal reasons actual culture media should be used to isolate *Neiserria gonorrhoeae* and *Chlamydia trachomatis*. In addition to bacterial cultures, a wet preparation should be performed on any vaginal discharge.

After the entire examination is completed, it is important to provide the patient with feedback and to describe your findings clearly to her. For patients who are premenarchal this is an opportunity to discuss puberty. Often, the anticipated time of menarche can be predicted on the basis of Tanner staging. And be sure to thank the patient for her cooperation.

THE ADOLESCENT PATIENT

The behavior that I observe in the waiting room helps me decide how to relate to adolescent patients. If the patient has come with her mother, I quickly assess how they are interacting in the waiting room. Their conversation and body language help me decide whether to initially interview the patient alone or accompanied by her mother. If the Mother appears to be comfortable, she may remain in the waiting room.

In some situations, you may choose to speak with the mother alone. She may have some specific thoughts to share with you, such as a family history of endometriosis or gynecologic malignancies. She may want to relate to you her anxieties about her daughter and issues such as sexual activity, contraception, or substance abuse.

Interviewing the Patient

Always remember that the teenager is the patient and the focus should be on her and her concerns. It is natural that an adolescent may regard your private conversation with her mother with feelings of suspicion and distrust. When talking with the patient alone, I usually can quickly defuse such feelings by telling her precisely what was discussed, quoting the Mother's words exactly. Recognizing what may be an all-too-familiar expression of her mother's concerns, the teenager usually replies, "Is that all she's worried about?!"

With the patient now somewhat more relaxed, I work hard to quickly establish a doctor-patient relationship that makes her feel comfortable and assures her that she can trust and confide in me. Therefore, I do not immediately launch into a discussion of the chief complaint. I begin by chatting with the teen in my office about something that is nonthreatening, such as school-related activities, friends, music, and clothing. Most of all, you have to be a good listener and nonjudgmental.

Do you have to look like a teenager to win confidence and be her doctor? No. You need to be yourself. For these patients, I usually wear my white lab coat. You can and should act as a role model. There is nothing wrong with an adolescent seeing the diplomas on your wall and aspiring to earn one of her own.

It is also important to discuss the principle of confidentiality with an adolescent patient, especially if you also happen to be her mother's gynecologist.[6] You need to take a general medical history, sexual and substance abuse history, and a gynecologic history. Your questions need to be phrased in a way that is developmentally appropriate for each patient, be she 13 or 19 years of age or somewhere in between. Do not assume that your patient is heterosexual. Ask about a history of sexual abuse, sexual assault, date rape, or possibly a physically abusive boyfriend.

Dealing with teen patients presents some common dilemmas. For example, the adolescent may present to your office accompanied by her mother with a chief complaint of dysmenorrhea. However, you need to keep in mind the strong probability that the teenager may have a much more important hidden agenda. If she is voluntarily sexually active, she may have been referred to you by her pediatrician to whom she has denied a history of sexual activity. Therefore, it is important that she trust you and that the two of you have a frank discussion of all the relevant facts. She may tell you that she wants birth control pills, but doesn't want her mother to know. What should you do? It is correct to respect her confidentiality and provide her with appropriate contraceptive counseling and technology. However, you might suggest that the two of you talk to the patient's mother about this. I usually approach this subject by asking the patient where she will keep the condoms, or diaphragm, or birth control pill package. What will she do if her mother accidentally discovers them? Will her mother really believe an excuse such as "they belong to a girlfriend"?

It should be noted that there are some limits to confidentiality. Specific legal statutes in each state designate health care professionals as mandated reporters and require reporting in certain situations. In general, confidentiality ends when the patient is placing herself or others in danger, when sexual or physical abuse is present or suspected, and when sexually transmitted diseases must be reported to local and state health authorities.

Examining the Patient

During the general physical and pelvic examination of adolescent girls, a chaperone should be present for a male physician. When the doctor is a woman, I believe she needs to decide on the basis of which option makes her more comfortable. In my own adolescent medicine practice, I usually do not have a chaperone for a routine gynecologic examination. In cases of alleged sexual abuse or sexual assault, the presence of a chaperone or assistant with every examiner is strongly recommended and should be documented in the medical record.

With teenagers, it is also important to explain the nature of the examination. You should review anatomy, terminology, and instrumentation with these patients using drawings, models, and diagrams. I show them the speculum and note that certain sounds are made as it is opened and closed, for example. You should stress to the patients that they are in control of the examination. As a result, discomfort should be minimal.

Start with a general physical examination. If the Mother did not leave your office during the interview, now is your opportunity to interview the adolescent alone. Reconfirm confidentiality and ask the questions that you may have withheld.

Obtain a weight, height, blood pressure, and urinalysis. Perform a breast examination to rule out the presence of any masses or galactorrhea. Record the Tanner stage of the breasts. This is an opportunity to discuss and teach breast self-examination. Perform an examination of the abdomen.

When performing the genital examination be sure to put the patient in control. With her in the lithotomy position, I prefer to place a cloth drape folded around her legs and directed inward to lie flat on her abdomen. This makes it easier for her to look down and observe. Offer her a mirror that she can hold to watch as you examine the vulva. Describe to her what you are doing. Remember to record the Tanner stage of the pubic hair and palpate for inguinal nodes. Select an appropriate speculum (Huffman, Pederson, or Graves) to view the vagina and cervix (see Figure 1-9). Be sure to let her check the temperature of the speculum by placing it against her thigh. As you spray the Pap smear slides, let her know that you are not spraying her. Perform a bimanual pelvic examination. At the conclusion of the examination thank her for being cooperative.

Laboratory Testing

With every sexually active adolescent's pelvic examination, test for *Neiserria gonorrhoeae* and *Chlamydia trachomatis* from the cervix. Always perform a wet preparation of any vaginal discharge. Perform yearly Pap smears for sexually active teenagers. Perform syphilis testing yearly, or more frequently if a patient has had a new sexual partner within the previous 3 months, is diagnosed with other STDs, has a history of cocaine/heroin use by herself or her sexual partner, or has a history of prostitution or survival sex. Apply liberal indications for pregnancy testing in all teenagers. Consider the need for hepatitis B testing for your teenage patients and council them on the availability of hepatitis B vaccine. Discuss and offer HIV antibody testing.

Post-Exam Counseling

After the examination is completed, have the patient dress and return to your office. Reassure her if the findings were normal or discuss the diagnosis if one was made. Provide her with literature on the diagnosis, contraception, breast self-examination, sexually transmitted diseases, AIDS, and condom use.[7] You should review birth control plans, condom use (have condoms available), laboratory tests done and how to get results, and when she should return. Remind her that you are accessible by telephone should she have any future questions or problems. Then, if appropriate, close the discussion with the mother (with patient's permission).

SUMMARY

All of us who care for patients routinely reach into our medical bags and pull out little collections of pearls and gems that we use to successfully diagnose and treat our patients. These tips, tricks, and tests will enhance your success when performing gynecologic examinations of pediatric and adolescent patients. Most examinations can be completed by being gentle, caring and, at each level, empowering the girl to participate in the examination. In the preadolescent and adolescent patient, the gynecologic examination should be an educational experience.

LITERATURE CITED

1. North American Society for Pediatric and Adolescent Gynecology. Controversies in pediatric and adolescent gynecology. NASPAG News. 1992;6(3):1.
2. Centers for Disease Control and Prevention. 1993. Sexually transmitted diseases guidelines. MMWR. 1993;42(No. RR-14):100.
3. Pokorny S, Storman J. Atraumatic removal of secretions from the prepubertal vagina. Am J Obstet Gynecol 1987;156:581.
4. Anderson C, Zeltzer L, Fanurik D. Procedural pain. In Schechter N, Berde C, Yaster M (eds). *Pain in Infants, Children and Adolescents.* Baltimore, Williams and Wilkins, 1993; pp 435–458.
5. Talbot C. The gynecologic examination of the pediatric patient. Pediatr Ann. 1986;15(7):501.
6. Blake J. Gynecologic examination of the teenager and young child. Obstet Gynecol Clin North Am. 1992;19(1):27.
7. *The Adolescent Obstetric-Gynecologic Patient.* ACOG Tech Bull 145. Washington, DC, American College of Obstetricians and Gynecologists, 1990.

CHAPTER 2

PEDIATRIC VULVOVAGINITIS

Janice Bacon, M.D.

INTRODUCTION

Complaints of vaginal discharge or vulvar irritation are common in a pediatric practice. Often the appearance of spotting or discharge in a child's panties or dysuria may be the first evidence of a problem. A premenarchal child with vulvovaginitis is often not seen by the obstetrician-gynecologist for initial care, but the patient may be referred as a last resort after a variety of treatments have been tried.

Familiarity with the normal physiology of the premenarchal genital tract and its variations is imperative for successful treatment of pediatric vulvovaginitis. This awareness allows development of an orderly plan for evaluation and therapy. Too often a problem may remain incompletely resolved or may become recurrent if its etiology is assumed and "shotgun" medications are prescribed. Some simple clues may also be overlooked if an incomplete examination is performed.

DEVELOPMENT OF THE GENITAL TRACT FROM BIRTH TO MENARCHE

Normal development of the premenarchal genital tract involves both anatomic and physiologic changes. The vulva, vagina, and genital organs undergo progressive changes from birth to puberty, and characteristic physiologic effects occur at various ages.

Anatomic Changes

In the infant, the vulva is smooth and hairless. The labia minora are prominent, falling over the opening of the vestibule. Vaginal length is approximately 4 cm and the ratio of cervix to uterus is 3:1. Hymenal diameter is approximately 4 mm. The ovaries are not palpable.

The developmental phase of childhood (ages 8 weeks to 7 years) can be called the "resting phase"—a time without endogenous hormone production and without exogenous stimulation from maternal hormones. The vestibule is poorly protected by the thin labia minora and flattened labia majora. The introital diameter is approximately 5 mm and the vagina is 4–5 cm in depth. The uterus has a tubular shape, and the ratio of cervix to uterus is 2:1. The ovaries are located at the level of the pelvic brim and range in volume from 0.7 to 0.9 cc.[1]

As puberty approaches, the vagina lengthens to approximately 8 cm, the hymenal diameter increases to approximately 1 cm, and the labia fill out and thicken. The uterine fundus becomes enlarged in relation to the cervix and lower uterine segment (cervix to corpus ratio of 1:1). The ovaries, now in the pelvis, may be seen to have an increasing number of small follicles, and ovarian volume increases to 2–10 cc.[2]

Physiologic Changes

In utero, the infant is directly exposed to the maternal hormonal milieu. Maternal estrogen produces vaginal hypertrophy in the infant. The superficial layer of the vagina is composed of stratified squamous epithelial cells containing abundant glycogen. After birth, withdrawal of maternal hormones occurs. The desquamation of these cells along with mucus from the stimulated cervix accounts for the "physiologic" white discharge seen in the neonate. Nitrazine testing of this material reveals a pH of 5.5–7.0. Passage of the infant through the maternal cervix and vagina may allow colonization of the neonate's vagina and rectum with maternal organisms such as *Escherichia coli*, coagulase-negative *Staphylococcus*, and *Lactobacillus*.[3]

Placental hormonal effects decrease gradually over the first 6–8 weeks after birth. Coincident with this diminished maternal effect, a small amount of bleeding from endometrial shedding may occur. Vaginal pH increases to 6.5–7.5. The vagina of the infant becomes colonized with nonpathogenic flora.

Once all effects of maternal estrogen are diminished, the superficial layers of the vagina become thin, atrophic, and glycogen deficient. Throughout the childhood years this environment provides a genital epithelium that is smooth, thin, and readily traumatized. These tissues lack the antibodies that are present in the post-menarchal adolescent and adult female. Anatomic positioning of the vaginal opening close to the rectum and the absence of vulvar enlargement and pubic hair may increase the risk for vulvovaginal inflammation. Potential problems may be exacerbated by children's hygienic practices: wiping from back to front, sliding on play surfaces or off toilet seats, and scratching the area with dirty hands and nails. Clothing that is too tight or nonabsorbent and obesity also may provide an increased risk for vulvar irritation.

Knowledge of normal physiology is also important at puberty. Several months before menarche, a thin clear-to-white discharge may begin. This nonirritating leukorrhea is composed of desquamated vaginal cells and endocervical mucus. It is associated with rising estrogen levels in the adolescent. Continued hormonal stimulation produces thickening of the vaginal epithelium with development of rugations. Vaginal size increases, labia enlarge, and pubic hair develops. Vaginal flora takes on an adult composition with increased numbers of *Lactobacilli* and colonization with *Candida*, *Gardnerella*, and other organisms (Table 2-1).

Postpubertal vulvovaginitis should be considered in light of adult vaginal flora and

Table 2-1.   Common Cervicovaginal Flora

Aerobes
  Escherichia coli   *Staphylococcus epidermidis*
  Lactobacillus sp.   *Streptococcus* sp.
  Corynebacterium sp.   (group B, enterococcus, alpha nonhemolytic)
  Gardnerella vaginalis

Anaerobes
  Bacteroides sp.   *Peptococcus* sp.
  Veillonella sp.   *Peptostreptococcus* sp.
  Gaffkya anaerobia   *Lactobacillus* sp.
  Binidobacterium sp.   *Eubacterium* sp.
  Clostridium sp.

physiology. The onset of sexual activity adds the consideration of sexually transmitted diseases to the spectrum of etiologies of vulvitis, vaginitis, or both.

SIGNS AND SYMPTOMS

Specific complaints of vulvovaginal irritation vary with the child's age. Infants may be irritable or cry with voiding; toddlers may also rub and scratch the area or pull at their diapers. The older child may pinpoint symptoms to the vulva and note itching, dysuria, or burning. Some may complain of odor. Questioning an older girl may localize the site of dysuria to the vulva. Examination of the child's clothing may reveal spotting or discharge; an odor may be present. On inspection, the vulva may be swollen or red and excoriations may be present. In chronic or recurrent cases, labial adhesions may be present and the skin of the affected area may thicken.

Sometimes, vulvovaginitis develops as a progression of symptoms originating as a primary vaginitis with secondary involvement of the vulva due to chronic dampness or maceration. Other times, a primary vulvar disorder may ascend to involve the vagina.

HISTORY AND PHYSICAL EXAMINATION

An older child may accurately describe symptoms of vulvovaginal irritation, but with an infant or toddler a detailed history must be obtained from the parents. Other caretakers of the child (e.g., babysitters, daycare workers) should not be overlooked. In cases of potential sexual assault, an accurate social history of all adults who care for a child must be obtained. The physician should feel comfortable addressing the possibility of sexual assault since it is often an unspoken parental fear. The physician can also address questions concerning symptoms associated with prior assault such as abdominal-pelvic pain, enuresis or encopresis, altered behavior, nightmares, and excessive masturbation.

Pertinent topics to cover in the history include the following:

- Onset of symptoms and accurate description
- Associated illnesses or infections (respiratory, skin, urinary tract, gastrointestinal, ear)
- Past illnesses (intestinal parasites, skin and autoimmune disease)
- History of normal growth and development
- Detailed social history and review of systems

- New household pets
- Recent travel
- Favorite play sites (sandboxes may provide sites for contacting insects or stool from animals)
- New personal care products used (soap, bubble bath, perfumes, powders, deodorant)
- Allergies (including reactions to medications, personal care products, detergents, clothing and foods)
- Medications (those prescribed for other medical problems as well as all prescriptions and over-the-counter products used for the present symptoms)
- Exposure to medications in utero (diethylstilbestrol)

Because a complete history is so important, but may be lengthy to obtain verbally, an office questionnaire can be developed to cover most of these topics. This can be mailed to the family in advance or filled out in the waiting room. This allows the physician to review the subject but focus on specific areas.

Physical examination of the premenarchal child requires patience, gentleness, and organization. Individualization is important. Gather all items that could be needed into one convenient place. Do not hurry! For most cases, an in-office examination will be sufficient. Begin with an inspection of the child's diapers, panties, or other clothing, noting color and odor of discharge and any signs of bleeding. Perform a complete physical examination. Note any dermatologic changes. Allow the child to familiarize herself with the examiner. Visit with an older child and show all instruments to be used. Allow older children to hold instruments until needed, thereby "participating" in the exam. The examiner should be familiar with techniques for examining each age group and the variety of instruments available. For practitioners who do not handle a great number of these problems, keeping all needed items in a decorative basket will aid organization and speed. Needed items include gloves, q-tips and calcium alginate (urethral) swabs, a syringe, pediatric feeding tube and red rubber catheter, and light source. Culture medium should be handy. A mirror is useful for demonstrating self-genital exam or explaining anatomic findings to older adolescents.

Most cases of vulvovaginitis in the premenarchal child will not require visualization of the entire vagina and cervix, nor require a bimanual examination. All information may be obtained from a "mini-inspection" of the vulva and lower third of the vagina. Whichever position the child is placed in, separation of the buttocks laterally and downward will allow a close look at the vestibule and lower vagina. Dr. Jean Emans' recommendation of a knee-chest position, however, may allow the entire vagina and cervix to be seen with this method.[5]

A gentle rectoabdominal examination will allow evaluation of the pelvis and palpation of many firm foreign bodies (marker caps).

Specimens should be gathered in a systematic fashion and kept to the minimum required. Cotton swabs may be dampened in normal saline to reduce irritation, or specimens may be procured by a few drops of normal saline introduced into the vagina and retrieved with a pipette and syringe. Some specimens may serve more than one purpose (e.g., one swab may be used to plate out culture medium and then be placed

Table 2-2.   Outpatient Sedation

Local
  Topical Xylocaine gel
  Topical diphenhydramine (Benadryl) and Kaopectate
Oral
  Chloral Hydrate
Intravenous
  Promethazine hydrochloride (Phenergan)
  Meperidine (Demerol) and promethazine hydrochloride

in a few drops of saline for wet mount). Dr. Susan Pokorny has developed a "catheter within a catherer" technique for vaginal irrigation and simultaneous collection of multiple specimens.[6] Simple irrigation with a syringe and tubing is also effective.

Careful documentation of all genital findings is imperative especially if sexual assault is suspected. Specific anatomic landmarks such as the hymen, perineum, and perirectal areas may need to be mentioned. An absence of abnormalities, however, may simply be stated as such without making measurements of the hymen or introitus, because those values may be altered by the examiner's technique or child's position. Many states have specific collection protocols or kits to facilitate legally correct collection of specimens in suspected assault cases and to aid detailed documentation and chain of custody.

An older child or adolescent may require a speculum exam of the upper vagina and cervix. An office inventory of assorted sizes and shapes (small, medium, large Pederson or Graves speculums) permits selection of an instrument most compatible with patient comfort.

A fearful or uncooperative patient may preclude an adequate examination in the office setting without adjunctive measures. Sedation, local or systemic, may be helpful (Table 2-2). An examination under anesthesia is more prudent, however, than a combative child and may be preferred by examiners who have had little experience with pediatric patients. Anesthesia in the operating suite may indeed be preferable in cases of suspected assault when photographs are needed or colposcopy is appropriate. Whenever sedation is used, appropriate personnel and facilities for recovery or complications must be available.

DIFFERENTIAL DIAGNOSIS

Vulvovaginitis accounts for more than 70% of gynecologic complaints in the pediatric age group. It occurs primarily because of poor perineal hygiene combined with a vulnerable anatomic and hormonal status. However, because more serious pathologic conditions may be the cause, an extensive differential diagnosis may be considered (Table 2-3). Recent publicity about sexual assault of children has heightened awareness and must be considered in appropriate patients. Symptoms may be more easily considered by differentiating a primary vulvitis with secondary vaginitis from a primary vaginitis and associated vulvitis.[1]

Table 2-3. Causes of Pediatric Vulvovaginitis

Poor Perineal Hygiene	System Illness
Physical Factors	Upper respiratory/ear
Foreign body	Gynecologic
Contact dermatitis	Urologic
Allergic reactions	Autoimmune
Trauma	Dermatologic
	Gastrointestinal
	Nonsexually Transmitted Diseases
	Sexually Transmitted Diseases

Table 2-4. Treatment for Vulvovaginitis due to Poor Perineal Hygiene

Comfort measures
  Warm sitz baths
  Bland emollients (Vaseline, A-D ointment, Desitin, Balmex)
Topical steroids
Secondary Infection of Excoriations
  Broad-spectrum antibiotics
  Burow's solution compresses
  Saline or Aveeno baths
Recurrent or Persistent Disease
  Estrogen cream (topically bid × 14 days)

Poor Perineal Hygiene

Vulvitis secondary to poor perineal cleansing and fecal contamination is the most common cause of external genital irritation in premenarchal children. Vaginitis is a secondary phenomenon. Though frequently described as "nonspecific," Gram stain or culture of discharge may reveal *Staphylococcus, Streptococcus,* diptheroids, anaerobes, or coliform organisms. Less common are commensals such as *Hemophilus* or *Candida.*

Inspection of the area may reveal erythema or edema and specks of smegma or stool may be noted on the vulva or perineum. Excoriations may be present along with occasional secondary infection. Specimen collection for culture is unnecessary unless abuse or a concomitant problem is suspected, or the problem is chronic. If a vaginal culture is performed, the best specimen is from the upper vagina. The laboratory should be informed of the appropriate clinical history and instructed to look for a predominant organism. Otherwise, any findings may simply be reported as consistent with "normal flora." Preferred media include blood or MacKonkey agar. Chronic conditions may exhibit a crusty erythematosis border along the inner aspect of the labia majora.

Management is directed to altering the child's methods of cleansing (front to back) and explanation to parents of proper care. Table 2-4 lists various treatments for specific cases. Topical steroids may relieve pruritis, and sitz baths with warm water are helpful. Secondary infection may require antibiotics, and severe cases of weeping dermatitis may be helped with Burow's solution compresses (1:40), saline solution, or colloidal oatmeal (Aveeno) baths. Topical anesthetics and antihistamines are to be avoided because these agents may cause sensitization and irritation.[1]

Marked improvement should be noted within 2 to 3 days. Further evaluation and culture should be taken if the course is not improved. Persistent or recurrent cases may be managed with topical estrogen cream applied twice a day for 10–14 days. Vaginal spotting may occasionally be seen after completion of estrogen therapy or after prolonged use.

Foreign Body

The presence of a foreign body in the vagina produces a primary vaginitis. Classic presentation is a purulent, foul, blood-tinged discharge. Children able to provide some history may note placement or "loss" of an article in the vagina. An endless array of small objects may be placed into the vagina—primarily out of curious self-exploration. Most common, however, are toilet paper fragments, carpet fibers, marbles, safety pins, or pen caps. These findings in children 3–8 years of age are the most common. Firm objects may be palpable on rectal exam or visualized in the office mini-pelvic exam. Complete removal of paper fibers, however, may require vaginoscopy and exam under anesthesia. A wet preparation reveals sheets of white cells, and cultures are not specific or helpful.

Office removal of the object(s) is preferred. Irrigation with diluted Betadine or warm saline is excellent but may not always remove all small fiber bits. Irrigation with warm solution introduced through the introital opening without touching the hymenal edges can be easily accomplished with a 10″ or 12-mm pediatric catheter and is usually tolerated well. Initiating the infusion while placing the catheter may also aid tolerance. Antibiotics are unnecessary. A routine x-ray film is not appropriate for diagnosis; the radiation exposure is needless and most routine flat-plate views of the abdomen do not involve the vaginal length entirely. Diagnosis by x-ray may still require removal of the object and complete inspection of the vagina and cervix with anesthesia. Objects that remain in the vagina for prolonged periods may produce an erosion into the vaginal mucosa or papillary changes on its surface.

Contact Dermatitis and Allergic Reactions

Many chemicals may be irritating to a small child's perineum by producing a "chemical irritation." Infant diaper rash falls into the contact dermatitis category. Urine and bacteria from stool together produce ammonia and other chemical irritants. This problem is compounded the buildup of heat and moisture held close to the body by the outer plastic diaper layer or rubber pants. This contact dermatitis affects the convex skin surfaces with skin creases being spared. Symptoms include erythema, erosions or vesicles, and possible secondary infection—frequently candida.[7]

Household laundry products such as soap and detergent may produce a similar contact dermatitis from residuals in clothing or cloth diapers. Contact reactions also may be caused by allergies to bath products such as bubble bath, perfume, deodorant, or toilet tissue dyes. Changing one item at a time to hypoallergenic nonperfumed or noncolored products may pinpoint a specific etiology. Use of a bland superfatted, nonperfumed soap (e.g., Neutrogena, Dove, Lowila) may be the best approach.

Trauma

Most traumatic injuries to the child's vulva or perineum produce vaginal bleeding, with or without swelling, and noticeable lesions (straddle injuries). Hematoma formation with late drainage from an intravaginal site may present as a dark or bloody discharge. Thermal trauma may occur from hot metal furniture or toys, or the perineum may be injured by wooden splinters. Treatment consists of symptomatic measures.

Systemic Illness

Infectious diseases from many body sites may be transmitted to the vulva or perineum. A child's contaminated hands, or those of a caretaker, may provide the vector. Specific examples include ear infections, upper respiratory or throat infections, gastrointestinal upset, and skin disease.

Systemic illnesses with skin manifestations may also have vaginal lesions. These include measles, scarlet fever, chicken pox, diphtheria, or blood dyscrasias (leukemia).

Symptomatic measures for vulvar lesions may include warm sitz baths (oatmeal, sodium bicarbonate); pat dry or dry with cool hair dryer. Compresses of water or Burow's solution may be used. Air circulation (no panties when possible) should be promoted.

Respiratory Infection

Respiratory pathogens that may infect the vulva or vagina include group A beta-hemolytic *Streptococcus, St. pneumoniae,* and *Neisseria meningitidis.* This secondary vaginitis may present as a white, yellow, or even slightly green discharge. Overgrowth of any organism normally present in the vagina may produce an abnormal discharge or other symptoms and may occur in the presence of coexistent systemic illness or antibiotic therapy. Identification of the primary source of disease with appropriate antibiotic therapy will also treat the vaginitis.

Skin Diseases

Dermatologic diseases pose a variety of presenting symptoms, primarily of vulvitis. A key to diagnosis of many is looking for skin manifestations on other parts of the body, particularly on sites such as the scalp, around the ears, elbows and knees, and skin folds. Among these diseases are atopic dermatitis, seborrhea, psoriasis, pityriasis, and lichen sclerosus; many of these have an autoimmune basis. Allergies, including those to environmental substances and foods, should be carefully noted.

Systemic skin diseases may be easily diagnosed when first seen on other body surfaces. Appropriate treatment may control symptoms, and vulvar lesions may never occur. When the vulva is the presenting site, however, the correct diagnosis may be overlooked, and the initial appearance may be altered by trials of medications (e.g., psoriasis). Atopic dermatitis may cause a severe or persistent vulvovaginitis. Patients with seborrheic dermatitis, a fairly common problem, frequently have disease sites around the ears with crusting, erythema, and fissuring. Other associated skin signs include keratosis piloris (dry papules on lateral arms and thighs), prominent fissures under the eyes, or scalp flaking with erythematous edges.[8]

Gynecologic and Other Disorders

Specific gynecologic causes of vaginitis include neoplasms: sarcoma botryoides, gonadal stromal tumors, benign lesions, and congenital anomalies. The most common malignancy of the lower genitalia in small children is sarcoma botryoides (embryonal rhabdomyosarcoma). Nonmalignant lesions encompass polyps from various sites. Evaluation should be oriented towards the suspected etiology. Procedures for workup may be best performed under anesthesia with vaginoscopy or colposcopically directed biopsies. Adjuvant measures such as ultrasound provide helpful information without patient discomfort.

Chronic vaginitis with secondary vulvar irritation may occasionally be evidence of a fistula or an ectopic ureter[9] and requires radiologic evaluation. Urethral prolapse may present with vaginal bleeding or mass, but most cases resolve spontaneously. Chronic or recurrent cases may benefit from estrogen cream twice a day for 2–4 weeks; urologic consultation is needed if unresolved. Urinary tract infections may present with dysuria or hematuria. Urinalysis is diagnostic and appropriate antibiotics produce rapid cure. Upper urinary tract sources (e.g., glomerular disease) may occasionally be involved.

A variety of other disorders, including autoimmune diseases and Kawasaki's disease, may produce signs or symptoms of vulvitis with occasional secondary vaginitis. An ectopic ureter or Chrohn's disease may lead to abnormal vaginal drainage as well as a mullerian anomaly with abnormal outflow tract. Lichen sclerosus may appear in the perineal region as ivory or pink flat-top papules, which are several millimeters in diameter or coalesce into atrophic plaques.[10]

Nonsexually Transmitted Diseases

Though it is difficult to determine the mode of transmission for all infectious diseases, many can be routinely grouped as primarily sexually transmitted or primarily transmitted by physical contact. The presence of organisms that can be transmitted in either fashion must always draw the physician's attention to possible abuse with appropriate evaluation.

Common nonsexually transmitted infectious diseases producing vulvar lesions or symptoms with occasional secondary vaginitis include molluscum contagiosum, bacterial infections (e.g., *Shigella*), parasites (e.g., pinworms), poison ivy, *Hemophilus vaginalis* (*Gardnerella vaginalis*), and *Candida albicans*. Treatment for these diseases is summarized in Table 2-5.

Molluscum contagiosum is common in young children and is seen frequently on the inner thigh and groin areas. It appears as raised pink, nonpruritic papules, with a depressed center producing a "bull's eye." Spontaneous resolution may occur, or curettage can be used to remove lesions. Other treatments include topical application of podophyllin or trichloroacetic acid and cryotherapy.

Pinworms, a common cause of vulvar and perirectal pruritis may result in excoriations

Table 2-5.   Treatment of Nonsexually Transmitted Diseases That Can Cause Vulvar Lesions

Disease/Pathogen	Treatment
Molluscum contagiosum	Curettage, podophyllin, cryotherapy, trichloroacetic acid
Shigella	Trimetroprim/sulfamethoxazole, 40 mg/kg/d q6h po, 7 days
Pinworms	Pyrvinium pamoate, 100-mg tabs po (treat family contact)
Tinea versicolor	Antifungal cream, bid or tid, 2–3 weeks
Intertrigo	Antifungal powders, tid, 2–3 weeks
Poison ivy	Topical products for itching, Benadryl
	Burow's compresses for weeping lesions
Candida	Antifungal cream, tid, 7–10 days
Group A β-streptococcus	Penicillin VK, 125–250 mg, qid × 10 days
Haemophilus influenzae	Amoxicillin 20–40 mg/kg/d, 7 days

and secondary infection. Symptoms customarily result from the adult female worm exiting the rectum nocturnally and depositing eggs on the external skin. Vaginitis and purulent discharge may occur when the adult worm enters the vagina instead of reentering the rectum, and the worm itself may be noted in the vagina. The best diagnostic procedure is a nocturnal application of scotch tape to pick up eggs.

The most common enteric pathogen is *Shigella*. All three forms of *Shigella* may produce a vaginal discharge that may be purulent or blood-tinged. A history of recent diarrhea in the patient or family member is variable. Treatment for this bacteria consists of trimethoprim/sulfamethoxazole 40 mg/kg/d in divided doses every 6 hours orally for 7 days.[11] These organisms may be noted in epidemics locally.

Tinea versicolor and intertrigo may also be passed from one person to another by nonsexual physical contact. Tinea is caused by a fungus and is easily recognized by the more lightly pigmented areas with irregular borders that are present primarily on the trunk of the body. In black patients, these involved areas may be more darkly pigmented. Gentle scrapping and microscopic examination reveals fungal elements when potassium hydroxide (KOH) is applied. Treatment consists of a mild antifungal cream or lotion applied two to three times a day for 2–3 weeks. Intertrigo is a nonspecific inflammatory condition usually found in skin fold areas such as beneath an abdominal panniculus. The superficial skin is white due to the constant moisture. The skin fold becomes red and somewhat shiny in appearance. Either *Candida* or tinea may be present; these can be diagnosed by wet preparation and KOH. Treatment is directed at symptomatic care to reduce moisture, such as talcum powder and antifungal powders.

Poison ivy also may be spread by children's hands to vulvar areas. Again, treatment is symptomatic. Weeping and macerated lesions may be treated with Burow's soaks.

Hemophilus vaginalis may be part of the normal vaginal flora in some youngsters but also may be sexually transmitted. Some infections with *H. vaginalis* are asymptomatic. Although this organism prefers the higher estrogen content of the postmenarchal vagina, colonization of an infant from birth due to contact with an infected maternal vagina is possible. The incidence of colonization, however, may be higher in children with a history of sexual abuse. Examination for physical signs of abuse and evaluation for traditional sexually transmitted diseases must be considered. Broad-spectrum antibiotics, such as ampicillin or metronidazole at 10–30 mg/kg/d in divided doses for 1 week are the treatments of choice.[6] Diagnosis is made by wet mount or by the production of a characteristic amine odor when KOH is added to the sample.

Candida also may be transmitted sexually and nonsexually. Like *Hemophilus,* this fungus prefers the more estrogenized vagina, with its higher glycogen level, of the older girl. However, *Candida* may be an agent of secondary invasion after other causes of vaginitis or vulvitis. Newborn infection may result from contact with the colonized maternal vagina, and risk of infection is enhanced by the presence of diapers. *Candida* infections may also be seen in older patients with diabetes mellitus, recent antibiotic use, or immunosuppression. Development of thrush may be spread to trunk and genitalia, especially when a pre-existing disease (intertrigo, eczema, seborrhea)[6] is present. Symptoms vary from mild erythema and pruritis, to intense scratching with excoriations, vesicles, weeping lesions, and satellite lesions. Borders of diseased areas are irregular. Chronic infection may produce skin thickening and discoloration. Treatment for mild cases is easily accomplished with antifungal cream (Desitin, Mycolog, Nystatin, miconazole), but severe cases may also require antibiotics for secondary infections. Symptomatic measures include sitz baths and air drying.

Sexually Transmitted Diseases

Although the hygienic habits of small girls may allow transmission of organisms traditionally considered transferred by sexual contact, the possibility of abuse must be strongly considered when these organisms are found in children. When possible, a close family history and evaluation of family members may provide additional evidence. Appropriate social service agencies must be notified. Diseases in this category include trichomoniasis, gonorrhea, chlamydia, syphilis, herpes, and condylomata acuminata. If abuse is suspected, the presence of organisms less frequently considered sexually transmitted (e.g., *Candida, Gardnerella, Mycoplasma, Ureaplasma*) must be considered in this light. The diagnosis of any sexually transmitted disease must prompt consideration of testing for others, including HIV. Table 2-6 summarizes treatment for sexually transmitted diseases.

Trichomonas, like *Candida* and *Hemophilus,* prefers the high estrogen content of the vaginal epithelium after puberty. The usual mode of transmission is sexual, but the organism may occasionally be acquired from swimming pools, wet towels, etc. Classic presentation of this primary vaginitis is a frothy green-yellow discharge, but the presence of other organisms may alter this appearance. Wet mount examination is the most specific method of diagnosis. Metronidazole has been the mainstay of treatment and may be given to children in doses of 10–30 mg/kg orally in three divided doses for 1 week.

Gonococci are occasionally transmitted to prepubertal children by close nonsexual contact or fomites; however, sexual abuse is the foremost means of transmission. Infection may be asymptomatic, but vulvovaginitis with copious purulent discharge, pruritis, labial swelling, and dysuria, is more common. Several methods of diagnosis are available. Gram's stain is a good preliminary study, but culture or monoclonal antibody assay (Gonozyme®) is best. Cultures should also be taken from oral and rectal cavities as the history suggests. Therapy includes a single dose of ceftriaxone 125 mg or 50 mg/kg intramuscularly once or oral amoxicillin 50 mg/kg (maximum 3 g). Each is given with probenecid 25 mg/kg orally (maximum 1 g). Penicillin-allergic patients may be treated with spectinomycin single dose 40 mg/kg orally (maximum 2 g). Tetracycline may be used in children older than 8 years at a dosage of 40 mg/kg orally (maximum

Table 2-6.   Treatment of Sexually Transmitted Diseases

Disease	Treatment	Dosage	Route	Days
Trichomoniasis	Metronidazole	10–30 mg/kg/24h dose, q6h	po	7–10
Gonorrhea	Ceftriaxone	125 mg,	im	
	or Spectinomycin	40 mg/kg	im	1
Children >45 kg		Adult regimen		
Children >age 8	Also treat for chlamydia empirically			
Alternate for older children:	Ceftriaxone	125 mg, single dose	im	
Penicillin-allergic	Spectinomycin	40 mg/kg, single dose	im	
Alternate for penicillin-allergic older children:	Tetracycline	40 mg/kg, single dose	im	
Chlamydosis	Erythromycin	50 mg/kg/24h, q6h	po	10
	or Erythromycin ethyl succinate	40 mg/kg/24h, q6h	po	7–10
	or Trimethoprim— sulfa methoxazole	20 mg TMP/kg/24h 100 mg SMX/kg/24h, qh6	po	7–10
Children 7–8 years	Doxycycline	100 mg, bid		7
Older children	Tetracycline	25–50 mg/kg/24h, q6h	po	7–10
Syphilis	Benazthine penicillin	50,000 U/kg, single dose	im	
Penicillin-allergic	Erythromycin or tetracycline	(doses above)	po	15
	Latent disease of unknown duration—double length of treatment			
Condyloma	Podophyllin (small lesions only), trichloroacetic acid, cryotherapy, laser treatment			
Herpes	Symptomatic care: Sitz baths, Burow's compresses, analgesics Secondary infection: broad-spectrum antibiotics			

2 g/day) in four divided doses for 1 week. Culture and therapy of all contacts must be carried out with follow-up and "test of cure" studies. If sexual assault is suspected, testing for gonorrhea or Chlamydia requires culture rather than other methods because no false-positives are possible with cultures.

Chlamydia, long recognized in pediatrics for its important role in inclusion conjunctivitis of the newborn and pneumonitis in infants, has also been noted as a cause of urethritis and vulvovaginitis in prepubertal children. This organism is associated with gonococcal infections, but it may be diagnosed with or without symptoms as a pathogen. Nonsexual modes of transmission are known including exposure of a newborn to an infected maternal cervix/vagina or, more commonly, transmission from conjunctival infections to the genital tract. When perinatal infection occurs, it is usually gone within 12–18 months after birth, although rare infants remain culture-positive up to 29 months.[10] If, however, a child has been treated with any broad-spectrum antibiotic (erythromycin) since birth, *Chlamydia* should not be present. Diagnosis is available by culture with McCoy cells after appropriate transport media or by monoclonal antibody assay (Chlamydiazyme®, Abbott Pharmaceuticals). This organism is capable of infecting the atrophic squamous cell epithelium of the prepubertal vagina causing a true vaginitis. This is contrasted to the preference for columnar epithelium in adults with endocervical infection. Treatment includes erythromycin, sulfonamides, or tetracycline for children over 8 years of age. Evaluation for other sexually transmitted diseases, particularly gonorrhea, must be done.

Syphilis is most serious in pediatric patients if it is congenital. Acquired forms, which may result from sexual assault, can have a clinical presentation similar to that of adults. The primary lesion (chancre) develops 10 days to 6 weeks after infection. The single, painless papule evolves into a 2- to 22-mm ulcer with a clean base and indurated edges. Its serum contains many spirochetes and diagnosis may easily be made by dark-field examination. Untreated cases progress to the secondary stage after 6 months, with the classic macular or papular skin disease characteristically found on palms and soles. Without treatment, 33% of patients develop tertiary disease 5–30 years later. A venereal disease research lab (VDRL) or rapid plasma reagin (RPR) test is adequate screening in the absence of lesions and must be repeated at 6–8 weeks after a suspected assault. Treatment consists of a single dose of Benzathine, penicillin G, 50,000 U/kg (maximum 2.4 million U), given intramuscularly. Injections should be repeated weekly for up to 3 weeks for latent disease of unknown duration. Penicillin-allergic children over 8 years of age may be treated with erythromycin or tetracycline in divided doses four times a day for 15 days. It should be kept in mind that the prevalence of syphilis is frequent in male homosexuals or after sexual assault by males.

Herpes type I or II may be sexually transmitted. Children usually present during the primary infection. An accompanying fever or groin lymphadenopathy may be present. Positive cultures are more likely if blisters are unroofed and the fluid within sampled. Lesions of the vagina or cervix may produce a discharge. Symptomatic relief may be attained with sitz baths and topical bland emollients (Vaseline). Classic, extremely tender, "blisterlike" vesicular lesions or ulcers in genital areas signal the possibility of sexual abuse. Acyclovir in oral or intravenous forms has not been used for herpes in pediatric patients, but adolescents may be given adult dosages of 200 mg orally 3–5 times a day while lesions are present. Topical Acyclovir cream may be helpful as well. Serologic testing generally is reserved for specific instances to determine whether the type I or II herpes simplex virus is present.

Like other sexually transmitted diseases, condylomata acuminata, caused by human papilloma virus, can be transferred by close contact or maternal transmission at birth; however, its presence should alert the physician to possible sexual abuse. Condylomata acquired at birth frequently is still present at 6–8 months of age and may be found up to 24 months of age but rarely longer. Some reports note transmission of viral types not usually on the genitalia of small infants from the hands of caretakers. Lesions generally have a papillary appearance or flat cauliflower form. Diagnosis of vulvar involvement can be made by visual inspection. Complete examination of the vagina and cervix is required, and anesthesia may be needed. Laser ablation is most frequently employed, especially if a number of lesions are present. When only a few lesions are present, they may be treated medically with bi- or trichloroacetic acid with symptomatic care by sitz baths and emollients. The child should be evaluated for other vaginal pathogens. Follow-up visits must be performed several times during the ensuing 6–12 months to treat any subsequent disease. Viral typing may be indicated especially if congenital etiology rather than assault seems likely.

LABIAL AGGLUTINATION

Irritation and inflammation from any vulvitis and/or vaginitis may produce labial adhesions. The presence of a midline raphe should prevent confusion with ambiguous genitalia. The labia minora adhere frequently from posterior areas first, then extend anteriorly. Most children are asymptomatic, and 80% resolve spontaneously in 1 year. Symptomatic children may complain of pain with activity, recurrent urinary tract infections, or an abnormal urinary stream maybe noted.

The most effective therapy for labial agglutination is estrogen cream applied to the vulva each evening for 2 weeks. Prolonged therapy may result in withdrawal bleeding when therapy is discontinued or produce breast swelling or tenderness. The patient's mother should gently separate the labia as much as possible. Surgical separation may be needed and, if performed, should be used in conjunction with postoperative estrogen cream for 2 weeks to promote healing. Occasional withdrawal spotting may be noted after the estrogen cream is discontinued. Cleansing of the vulva is imperative. All environmental irritants (e.g., bubble bath) must be eliminated. Recurrent episodes of agglutination may be associated with chronic dermatologic disorders. Small posterior agglutination may occur even after treatment but requires no further action if asymptomatic.

SUMMARY

Vulvovaginitis is a common, easily managed problem in most prepubertal girls. A broad differential diagnosis must be considered, particularly if sexual abuse is a possibility or the problem is recurrent. Familiarity with the potential causes and presentations will improve physicians' ability to pinpoint the etiology and treat patients expediently. Treatment in the prepubertal age group with antibiotics requires a familiarity with pediatric dosing for various antibiotics. Recurrences of sexually transmitted diseases should make one suspect the possibility of sexual abuse.

LITERATURE CITED

1. Gidwani GP. Approach to evaluation of premenarchal child with a gynecological problem. Clin Obstet Gynecol 1987;3:643.
2. Fleischer AC, Shawker TH. The role of sonography in pediatric gynecology. Clin Obstet Gynecol 1987;3:735.
3. Gerstner GJ, Grunberger W, Boschitsch E, et al. Vaginal organisms in prepubertal children with and without vulvovaginitis. Arch Gynecol 1982;231:247.
4. Miller JM, Pastorek JG. The microbiology of premature rupture of the membranes. Clin Obstet Gynecol 1986;29:740.
5. Emans SJ, Goldstein DP. The gynecologic examination of the prepubertal child with vulvovaginitis: use of the knee-chest position. Pediatrics 1980;65:758.
6. Pokorny S. Prepubertal vulvovaginopathies. Obstet Gynecol Clin North Am 1992;1939.
7. Altchek A. Vulvovaginitis, vulvar skin disease, and pelvic inflammatory disease. Pediatr Clin North Am 1981;2:397.
8. Altchek A. Common problems in pediatric gynecology. Compr Ther 1984;10:19.
9. Kingsbury A. The clinical importance of vaginal discharge in childhood. Aust NZ J Obstet Gynecol 1984;24:135.
10. Friedman E. *Vulvar Disease.* Philadelphia, WB Saunders, 1983.
11. Vanderen AM, Emans SJ. Vulvovaginitis in the child and adolescent. Pediatr Rev 1993;14(4):141.

CHAPTER 3

PEDIATRIC SEXUAL ABUSE

Susan F. Pokorny, M.D.

INTRODUCTION

Evaluating a child for possible sexual abuse is not straightforward. These evaluations are frequently biased by the perceptions, experiences, clinical practices, and resources of the evaluator. Some cases are simple and others complex. Even some straightforward cases are not as simple as they may initially appear.

I recall, for example, a seemingly straightforward case involving a 6-year-old black girl who had physical findings and gave a good history. The girl "believed" she had been touched in the genital region by a male lifeguard who had jumped into the public swimming pool and pulled her to the side. She later reported that he had put his "cold" finger into her vagina while pulling her along. The child promptly reported the incident to a staff counselor. The mother was called and took the child, still in her wet bathing suit, immediately to a children's hospital; after a 4-hour wait, an intern assigned to the child abuse team examined the child. This intern noted erythema of the vulva and no hymen. The mother was informed that there were definite findings of abuse. Three days later, an experienced child abuse physician examined the child and noted "no erythema" and a "low rim of normal hymenal tissue." The child abuse team strongly supported prosecution of the case based on the initial finding of genital erythema and the child's comments about genital touching.

Unfortunately, the medical team were not aware that the child had previously been sexually abused and been counseled after that incident to immediately report other attempts at molestation. They also were not aware that the lifeguard had jumped into the pool not to assist the child, but rather to discipline her. She had pushed another child and had been told to go to the "timeout" area; instead she had jumped into the deep end of the pool. The medical team also did not know that two other lifeguards, in close proximity, gave sworn depositions that after seeing their colleague jump into the pool, they had carefully watched his entire performance, thinking he was attempting a rescue and might need their help.

During the time that the case was being prosecuted, the mother was encouraged to keep the child in therapy and "great emotional suffering" occurred, not to mention expense. However, several things about this case suggest that abuse did not occur:

1. The close eyewitness accounts of the "episode" made abusive behavior unlikely.

2. The erythema of the vulva was most likely due to an unestrogenized child having to sit in a wet bathing suit for 4–6 hours.

3. The touch that the child described as "cold" was probably a cold bleb of water trapped between the child's genitals and bathing suit. Stretch trauma, which would have occurred if the large male lifeguard's digit had gone into a petite 6-year-old's vagina, causes a "burning" sensation.

4. The child's prior history of abuse and subsequent counseling, as well as the child's anger at the lifeguard, would explain the child's behavior and her interpretation of her experience.

I present this case to illustrate the impact of referral patterns. If the child had seen her regular physician, it is possible the situation just described might have had a more saluatory outcome. The private physician might have obtained more details about just exactly what had happened and proceeded more cautiously if he understood the child was being disciplined. The child's own physician would also most likely have known about her prior history and abuse counseling. In contrast, an intern assigned to the sexual abuse team, when asked to perform a forensic genital examination on a child sent to an emergency room, is going to interpret physical findings and comments as compatible with abuse.

THE ROLE OF PRIMARY CARE PHYSICIANS

It goes without saying that physicians must be comfortable and competent in performing genital examinations on children of all ages (see Chapter 1) before they start doing such examinations to look for physical findings of sexual abuse. Currently many physicians feel uncomfortable in performing genital examinations, particularly on survivors of sexual abuse. In 1993, there were 6000 reported cases of childhood sexual abuse in Santa Clara County, California; only 600 hundred of these cases had physical examinations at the medical center that conducts the vast majority of specialized examinations. In other words, "the site of the crime" was not inspected in close to 5400 of the 6000 cases; a major opportunity to substantiate the "outcry" of the sexual abuse survivor was missed the majority of the time. The importance of medical evidentiary examinations is underscored by a study of suspected abuse cases occurring in New York in 1992.[1] When the medical community was involved in reporting and/or evaluating cases (13% of the total), the final determination was that evaluation/investigation was "indicated" 40% of the time. In contrast, when the medical community was not involved (87% of total cases), evaluation/investigation was "indicated" only 29% of the time.

Primary care physicians have the advantage of knowing a possible abuse victim's life history. They also are likely to see the child more quickly and in a less anxiety provoking situation than present in a crowded emergency room. Private physicians also can maximize therapeutic encounters with the child due to continuity of care. When anatomic findings are difficult to interpret or are unusual, they can consult with pediatric gynecologic experts.

Currently however, we have to support the "sexual abuse experts" and their programs for several reasons. Many primary care physicians refuse to get involved in sexual abuse cases. As a group, the experts are examining the thorny issues of conflicts between the medical community and the legal system such as subpoena interruption of practice profiles and lack of reimbursement for evidentuary examinations and for court time. These experts also are able to analyze the clinical findings that could be used to substantiate the child's outcry.

PHYSICAL EVIDENCE OF ABUSE DENIED BY THE CHILD

The majority of childhood sexual abuse evidentiary evaluations are initiated because of the child's verbal or behavioral "outcry." A difficult situation occurs when the physician "discovers" strong physical evidence of abuse (e.g., a positive GC culture or a genital laceration entering the vagina through the hymen) and the child denies injury or a fall. In such situations, charges are rarely filed unless the child gives a statement of abuse.

I recall an 8-year-old girl who was brought to me by her mother who had noticed blood clots on the child's bedding and had felt that the child was much to young to be starting her menstrual period. Before bringing the girl to me, the mother gave the history that the child had adamantly denied any injury; when I evaluated the child in my office, she seemed quite composed and denied that there had been any injuries or fall the preceding day. She also showed no signs of estrogen stimulation such as breast buds. However, when I examined the child's genital area fresh abrasions and ecchymoses were quite apparent; one of the linear abrasions extended from the vestibule into the posterior wall of the vaginal floor. Closer inspection revealed that only hymenal remnants were present. The hymenal remnants indicated to me that there had been chronic abuse or chronic stretch trauma. The fresh ecchymoses and abrasions clearly indicated that some traumatic event had occurred within the past 24 hours. However, upon showing the child these areas on her genital area with a hand-held mirror, she again adamantly denied that anybody had touched or injured her.

Given this scenario, I informed the mother that I believed someone was harming her daughter and requested that she wait in my office until the child protective services had been notified and could come to the office to assist us with further management. While we were waiting for child protective services, the child's father arrived and was so verbally abusive to the staff that security was immediately notified. However, before security could arrive the father took the mother and the child home. Over the next several hours, the time it took for child protective services to obtain police escort to go to the home, the child changed her story and stated that she had been wrestling with her brother and had accidentally fallen on his finger. Nevertheless, due to my strong conviction that an injury had occurred that the child was denying, protective services removed the child into protective custody for a 2-week period of time. At the court hearing, the child still adamantly denied that any injury had occurred in her home, and for this reason she was returned to her home. To my knowledge no further actions were taken in terms of investigating this family or in protecting this child.

BALANCING HISTORY AND PHYSICAL FINDINGS

The examining physician needs to take into account why he or she is evaluating a particular child. Is it for signs and symptoms that would include abuse in the differential? Is it for signs and symptoms for which abuse is highly likely? Or is it for signs and symptoms for which others are adamant that abuse has occurred?

When the signs and symptoms for which the child is brought to the physician would include sexual abuse in the differential, such as prepubertal genital bleeding, the history and the evolution of the signs and symptoms must be emphasized to differentiate a medical illness with genital or rectal pain, infection, or bleeding from childhood sexual abuse. On the other end of the spectrum, sexual abuse will be highest on the differential if the history includes behavioral abnormalities such as precocious sexual behaviors, or the physical findings noted at the time of the evaluation include sexually transmitted diseases or anal/genital wounds compatible with assault. When a child has been thought to have been sexually assaulted but there has been no specific "outcry," the history and physical are equally weighted and should be meticulously recorded.

Examiner biases can be dangerous when an agency sends the child for a medical evidentiary evaluation. This is a very dangerous situation for the clinician because physical findings tend to be emphasized and less effort is taken to understand the overall life situation of the child that might explain observed physical findings. Once I was requested to see a child on an emergency basis as she was being transported from one hospital to a children's hospital via ambulance. All that was written on the referral sheet was "sexual assault," and the child clearly had a significant injury in her genital area. There was a large amount of blood in the genital area, and the child seemed to be in early stages of hemodynamic instability. An intravenous line was started, and she was prepared for the operating room. There was a large vestibular laceration on the right side, and the entire right perineum was becoming discolored. Closer inspection revealed an intact hymen to the left of the large laceration, however, and vaginoscopy showed an intact vaginal canal. This seemed to be an unlikely injury from a sexual assault, as the force of the sexual assault would have entered the vaginal canal, whereas this injury was immediately adjacent to but to the right of the vaginal canal extending into the ischial rectal fossa approximately 6 inches. The wound was debrided, drains were placed, and an intraoperative x-ray revealed that the child had six pelvic fractures, four on the right side and two on the left. An exploratory laparatomy revealed that the child had a large right sidewall expanding retroperitoneal hematoma. A diverting colostomy was performed to help with the hygiene of the large perineal wound.

The mother was the only historian for the child. Most significantly the emergency technicians had noted no blood in the parking lot location where the mother stated that she had found her daughter lying on the ground; the only blood stains observed were on the couch in the family living room and on the mother's clothing. Two weeks into the child's hospitalization, the mother changed her story and stated that the child had been struck by a car. Again this history seemed unlikely because there were no other abrasions or wounds on the child's body except in the perineal/pelvic area. With support, this traumatized family eventually revealed that the child had been crushed by the bumper of an automobile against the building when her undocumented illegal alien uncle had accidentally placed the car into forward instead of reverse, thereby crushing the child's pelvic bone between the car and the apartment building. This crush trauma had initiated a massive retroperitoneal hematoma due to the pelvic fractures. This hematoma did not rupture in the parking lot, explaining the absence of blood there. Due to its tremendous size the hematoma ruptured through the vulvar tissues after the mother had carried the child to the couch where the emergency technicians ultimately found her. With evacuation of the hematoma, the large vestibular laceration was created. This case illustrates the importance of ascertaining whether any genital wound discovered is compatible with the history given. If on face value this child had been signed off as a sexual assault survivor, she tragically would have been removed from a loving and caring home.

The history recorded by the physician is very important in childhood sexual abuse cases. It is very important that the physician understand the "hearsay rule." For example, when the child has discussed the abusive episode with a neighbor or a friendly acquaintance, an account of the conversation by the friend is not allowed in a court of law under what is called the "hearsay rule." On the other hand, because the patient-physician relationship is a privileged and confidential relationship, what a child says to a physician has in the past been allowed as evidence in a court of law. This rule places the burden upon the physician to be extremely careful to "not put words into the child's mouth." Statements by the child must be recorded in the medical record verbatim and in the words that the child would use. During questioning of the child, statements should be given in an open-ended manner so as not to lead or cajole the child into saying what the physician would expect the child to say. "Tell me more" and "then what happened" are examples of acceptable open-ended statements or queries.

When signs or symptoms in the medical history raise suspicions about possible childhood sexual abuse, I typically share my concerns with the parent(s) or guardian who brought the child for the medical evaluation. One way I explain to parents the importance of further evaluation for possible sexual abuse is to share with them the following scenario. If I saw a suspicious growth on their child's perineum and decided not to biopsy it, but rather said "why don't we just have her come back in a year or so and see if it's malignant or not," they wouldn't tolerate my management of that condition. By the same token, if I am suspicious of possible childhood sexual abuse but do nothing, I am guilty of mismanagement. When presented in this manner, the vast majority of parents and guardians are more than ready to comply with further evaluation. Informing a parent that their child may have been sexually abused is as traumatic as if you had told them that their child had a malignancy, and one must be ready with appropriate support, information, and reassurance.

CONDUCTING AN EVIDENTIARY MEDICAL EXAMINATION

The evidentiary medical examination is fairly simple. The health care professional needs to document sexually transmitted diseases, document and describe perineal injuries (especially with reference to disruptions of the hymen), and possibly collect medical forensic evidence as required by rape kits. Rape kits are composed of protocols for obtaining forensic data; they vary in different areas of the country, but basically are very much the same. The examiner simply follows the protocols. A rape kit is a tool for documenting findings at the site of the crime; therefore, the transfer and storage of the materials collected must be handled so that the medical provider can state that nobody could have tampered with this evidence. Most protocols require that specimens placed in a rape kit be properly labeled and initialed.

In the vast majority of childhood sexual abuse cases, however, rape kits are not indicated because the child's outcry occurs weeks or months after the alleged assault. For this reason, there would be no debris on the child's body that would substantiate her story. If there is a possibility that sexual contact might have occurred recently, then a rape kit protocol should be followed on a young child. With adults, if the assault occurred more than 72 hours before the examination, a rape kit is not indicated, as no debris would remain on the survivor's body. However, in a prepubescent child without hormonal stimulation, there is minimal vaginal discharge and minimal leukorrhea for purging the body of any intravaginal semen or sperm. Because the child's vagina is a relatively inert space, sperm and semen may be detectable in a prepubescent vagina for a period greater than 72 hours. I have extended the use of rape kits to at least a week in the prepubescent unestrogenized child. These rape kits should be performed in an atraumatic manner; if there is a strong possibility that debris substantiating the child's outcry is present but the child is uncooperative, an examination under anesthesia is indicated. It is important to keep in mind that a medical evidentiary examination should be atraumatic.

It should be noted that foreign objects in the vagina of a prepubescent child have many of the signs and symptoms similar to those of a sexual assault survivor. The posterior rim of the hymen is frequently irregular and intermittent spotting or vaginal bleeding often occurs in both situations. Because of the dependent position of the vaginal introitus, it is conceivable that many foreign objects are expelled with either the forces of gravity or when the patient performs a valsalva maneuver. I have recently reported on some papillary projections in the vaginal vault associated with an expelled foreign object that the examiner should look for at the time of vaginoscopy. The presence of such papillary projections might suggest that further work-up for sexual abuse is unnecessary. Clearly, additional studies are needed in this area.

Speculum examinations should not be performed on prepubescent children. If vaginoscopy needs to be performed, use of an irrigating endoscope is strongly recommended. The small diameter of the endoscope will not traumatize the unestrogenized vaginal walls or the hymenal rim. After the vagina has been lavaged with the irrigating fluid, the vulvar tissues can be gently squeezed against the endoscope, allowing the irrigating fluid to distend the vaginal vault so that it can be seen in its entirety including the cervix at the apex.

EVALUATION OF THE FINDINGS

An area of great confusion for physicians is matching the history of a genital injury with those of the genital wounds observed. My colleagues and I have reported on 32 cases that involved history of a genital injury and visualization of an acute genital wound.[3] In this series, only three of the *symmetric* perineal injuries that *transected* the hymen were *not* related to sexual assault. In all the other cases with a symmetric midline genital injury transecting the hymenal tissues, sexual assault was the cause.

Other strong physical evidence of sexual assault are hymenal caruncles. In the adult

TABLE 3-1. Consistent But Not Diagnostic Findings for Childhood Sexual Abuse*

Chafing, abrasions, or bruising of the inner thighs and genitalia
Scarring, tears, or distortions of the hymen
Decreased amount or absence of hymenal tissue
Scarring of the fossa navicularis
Injury to or scarring of the posterior forchette
Scarring or tear of the labia minora
Enlargement of the hymenal opening

*Italicized words are action descriptive and misleading.
Source: Adapted from R Krugman, JA Bays, D Chadwick, et al. Committee on Child Abuse and Neglect, American Academy of Pediatrics. Guidelines for evaluation of sexual abuse of children. *Pediatrics.* 1991;87:254.

physiologically mature female's body, hymenal caruncles occur after the delivery of an object the size of a term-sized infant's head.[4] In the unestrogenized prepubescent child, hymenal caruncles occur after the stretch trauma caused by an object the size of the adult erect phallus, as occurs in sexual assault. I have observed similar injuries in young girls who have had a large speculum placed in their vagina. It must be stressed that after the estrogen stimulation that occurs in the body beginning in puberty, significant and serious trauma can occur to the estrogenized hymen without permanent sequelae.

Premenarchal genital bleeding should raise the physician's suspicion of childhood sexual abuse. However, the clinician must be aware that there are common pediatric gynecologic problems such as urethral prolapse, lichen sclerosis, maternally transmitted condyloma accuminata, and vulvovaginitis that can cause premenarchal genital bleeding. Other less common pediatric gynecologic problems that cause premenarchal genital bleeding include hymenal tags, cervical polyps, and hematologic lesions such as hemangiomas and congenital telangiectases.

The Committee on Child Abuse and Neglect of the American Academy of Pediatrics has guidelines for the evaluation of sexual abuse of children.[5] Unfortunately, the terms used in these guidelines are "action descriptive" and therefore misleading (Table 3-1). For example, the description "scarring or tears of the hymen" might be described more appropriately with anatomic terms such as hymenal remnants or nubbins of tissue.

In evaluating suspected childhood sexual abuse cases, physicians should remember that some children are born with very low rims of hymenal tissue, and occasionally the vestibular rim is so prominent as to occasionally be confused with the hymen, which is more recessed into the vestibular vault and on the same plane as the urethra. In determining the amount of hymenal tissue present, the physician must be cognizant of the effect of estrogen on the hymen.[6] The clinician also needs to take into account that the hymenal opening is affected by the relaxation and position of the child and by the configuration of her hymenal tissues, as well as by the presence or absence of hymen variants such as a microperforate hymen.

SUMMARY

Evaluating a child for sexual abuse is not straight forward—some cases are simple and others complex. Understanding the intricacies of history taking is most essential. The primary care physicians have the advantage of knowing a possible abuse victim's life history. Most evidentiary evaluations are initiated because of the child's verbal or behavioral, "outcry". Examination bias can be dangerous when an agency sends the child for a medical evidentiary evaluation. The physical examination should be as gentle as possible. Other causes, than sexual abuses, must always be considered in the evaluation of the history and the findings. It is important for the physician to keep in mind that therapeutic efforts begin with your first contact with the child and that no procedures should be performed that would add to the trauma the child has already experienced.

LITERATURE CITED

1. Kerns DL, Terman DL, Larson CS. The role of physicians in reporting and evaluating childhood sexual abuse cases. In Behrman RE (ed). *The Future of Children: Sexual Abuse of Children.* Los Altos, Calif, 1994, The David and Lucille Packard Foundation; p. 122.
2. Pokorny SF. Long term intravaginal presence of foreign bodies in children: a preliminary study. J Reprod Med. 1994; 39(12):931.
3. Pokorny SF, Pokorny WJ, Kramer W. Acute genital injuries in prepubertal females. Am J Obstet Gynecol. 1992;166(5):1461.
4. Cunningham FG, McDonald PC, Gant NF, et al. Anatomy of the reproductive tract of women. In Cunningham FG, McDonald PC, Gant NF, Leveno KJ, Gillstrap LC (eds). *Williams Obstetrics.* 19th ed. Norwalk, Conn, Appleton & Lange, 1963; p. 60.
5. Krugman R, Bays JA, Chadwick D, et al. Committee on Child Abuse and Neglect, American Academy of Pediatrics. Guidelines for evaluation of sexual abuse of children. Pediatrics. 1991;87:254.
6. Yordan EE, Yordan RA. The hymen and tanner staging of the breast. Adolesc Pediatr Gynecol. 1992;5(18):76.

SUGGESTED READINGS

Emans SJ, Woods EF, Flagg NT, Freeman A. Genital findings in sexually abused, symptomatic and asymptomatic, girls. Pediatrics. 1987;79(5):778.
Medical evaluation of the child victims of sexual abuse. Muram D. Curr Sci. Vol 1, pgs 250–258, 1989;1:250.

GENITAL TRAUMA IN CHILDREN AND ADOLESCENTS

Janice L. Goerzen, M.D.

INTRODUCTION

Three major questions must be answered immediately when attending children with genital trauma on an emergent basis. Is resuscitation required? (Active bleeding, interference with local or system function, life threatening.) Is the trauma of genital or nongenital origin? (Gastrointestinal disorders such as polyps, fissures, and Meckel's diverticulum, genitourinary situations such as urethral prolapse, and any condition in the differential diagnosis for hematuria may present with what appear to be genital trauma.) Is the condition truly trauma of the genital tract or pathology masquerading as trauma?

If trauma is present, several causes are possible. Accidental lacerations, chemical or thermal burns, or fractures may produce genital trauma. Nonaccidental causes of genital trauma include abuse resulting from burns (hot stoves or bath), human bites, self or other induced foreign body, and mutilation (e.g., sunna, clitoridectomy, or infibulation). Iatrogenic causes of genital trauma include injuries from surgical cautery or laser, scalpel, or instrumentation. Corrosives such as podophyllum or trichloracetic acid can also contribute to this type of trauma.

Pathology affecting the genital system often is associated with injury from scratching or other direct injury to perineal lesions. Examples of such conditions are lichen sclerosis et atrophicus, dermatitis, eczema, psoriasis, infections caused by herpes zoster or genitalis and coxsacki B virus, molluscum, hemangiomas, and the full differential for nontraumatic vaginal bleeding.

HISTORY

At some point in the history or examination, the child should be seen alone to give her account of the trauma. Note, however, that younger children may not have developed

Table 4-1. Criteria for Surgical Treatment of Genital Trauma*

- Inadequate examination
- Psychologically better for child to do Examination Under Anesthesia (EUA)
- Vital signs unstable due to injury
- Laceration larger than 1.5–2.0 cm
- Active bleeding from wound
- Extension of injury through hymen and/or above the hymen
- Expanding hematoma or above the mons
- Hematuria or unable to void
- Pain not responding to conservative means
- Other injuries requiring surgical treatment
- Follow-up unreliable with inadequate examination

*Medical criteria are the opposite of these surgical criteria.

accurate concepts of time, place, or the complex relationships among adults. Because the child is often guilt ridden and or afraid about her experience, the physician must strive to get a complete history without making the child even more anxious. The parent or attendant will give most of the details. But the best approach for evaluating the possibility of abuse is to first question the child in a friendly way and then have the parent confirm her account.

Relevant questions to be addressed include the following:

- Who caused the injury? What was done? Where and how was the trauma inflicted? Were there any witnesses?

- Are there any other injuries?

- How much bleeding occurred and how big is the lesion? Is the lesion stable, increasing, or decreasing?

- Has the child passed urine since the traumatic incident?

- Was any foreign body passed by the child or other?

- Apart from the presenting trauma, What is the child's current and past health? Has she had previous emergency room visits or previous episodes of trauma?

- What allergies does the child have?

- When did she last eat and drink?

PHYSICAL EXAMINATION

A full physical examination is mandatory. In one case a ruptured spleen and bruised kidney were responsible for the "vaginal bleeding," which was actually hematuria detected when the child returned to the ward after repair of a fractured leg. Vital signs and weight are important.

The amount of bleeding, the size and rate of change of the lesion, and the other surgical criteria listed in Table 4-1 can assist in deciding whether an operative or conservative approach to care is indicated. The urethra, hymen, and lower third of the vagina can often be seen in the knee-chest position. The child can often be coaxed to help part labia and will frequently do it with more vigor and courage than the attending physician.

MANAGEMENT

Not all the criteria listed in Table 4-1 need be present for surgery to be warranted. However, a preponderance of medical criteria (opposite to the surgical criteria) would suggest that a conservative, medical approach is appropriate.

Surgical Management

I recommend the following guidelines for surgical management of genital trauma in children:

1. Carry out preoperative assessments as required. These might include hemoglobin, coagulation parameters, ultrasounds, x-rays, CAT scans.
2. Use anesthetic patches to establish intravenous for hydration. Child is kept NPO until assessment and/or surgery is completed.
3. Consider a general anaesthetic for surgery, as it often permits a better examination and results in less psychological trauma for the child.
4. Use an antibiotic if the injury is unclean. A tetanus shot may be needed depending upon the nature of the wound.
5. Perform a vaginoscopy, insertion of a urethral catheter and, if necessary, a cystoscopy. The best instrument for vaginoscopy is a pediatric cystoscope operated with running saline or water. Dry instrumentation is traumatic and does not offer as good a view, nor flush the vagina, as does wet examination. Perform a rectal examination.
6. Use a finer suture than that used for adults.

Lacerations extending past the hymenal ring can extend along the perivaginal fascia and into the retroperitoneal space. This is so especially if vaginal hematomas occlude the vagina. Utilize drains, packs, antibiotics, ultrasounds, and laparatomy as required. Follow vital signs and hemoglobin postoperatively, as the quantity of blood loss may not be reliable. Tie bleeding vessels, and suture the vaginal wall with figure of eight sutures. Large retroperitoneal hematomas usually result from rupture of the vessels above the pelvic floor. An artificial vaginal septum may result after vaginal surgery in the prepubertal child, and follow-up near menarche is advised.

Contusions above the clitoris or extending into the mons or above can extend even higher up and lead to necrotizing fasciitis. Antibiotic, pressure, and icepacks (wrapped to prevent skin damage) are helpful. If pressure dressings (poorly tolerated by most children) are necessary to prevent extension of the contusion, then the surgery may not have adequately controlled the bleeding from vessels. In contusion injuries, especially those sustained in motor vehicle accidents, the labia may receive a "smack" laceration on their medial surfaces. Expel clots and suture. An expanding labial laceration is also best treated by medial (vs lateral) incision into the labia. Deep sutures may be necessary to stop bleeding from the labial venous plexus.

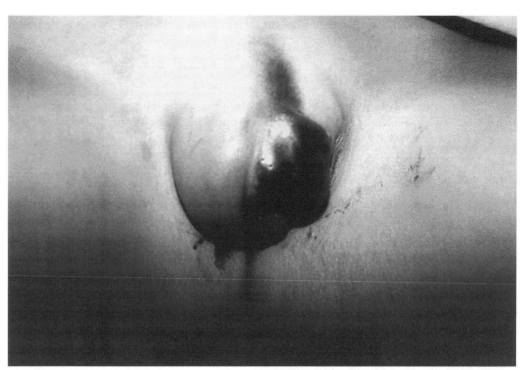

Vulvar hematoma in a prepubertal girl. (From the NASPAG PediGYN Teaching Slide Set. Photographic image courtesy of Marta C. Mendez, M.D.)

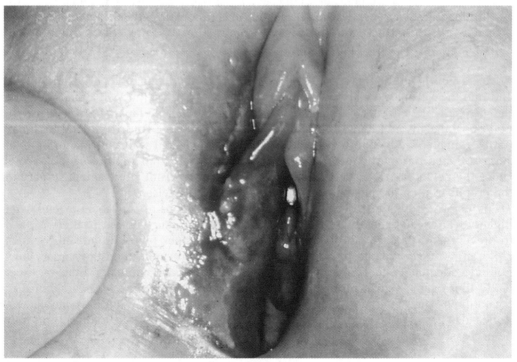

Acute straddle injury in a young child with a typical distribution of trauma. (From the NASPAG PediGYN Teaching Slide Set. Photographic image courtesy of Martin A. Finkel, D.O.)

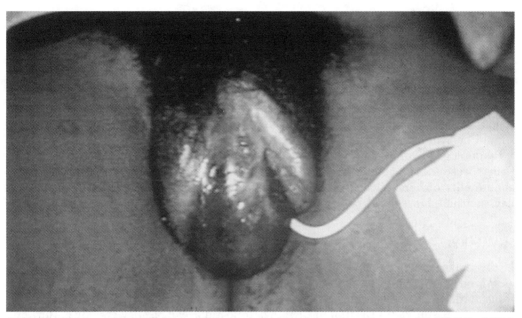

Vulvar hematoma in an adolescent. A foley catheter is in the urethra. (From the NASPAG PediGYN Teaching Slide Set. Photographic image courtesy of Diane F. Merritt, M.D.)

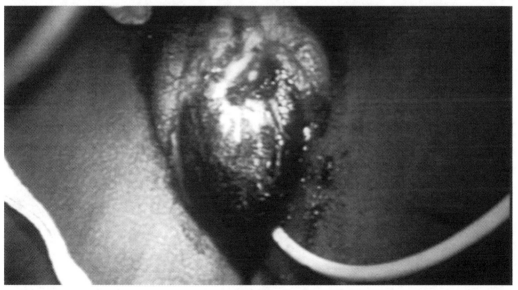

Tissue necrosis resulted as a consequence of inadequate drainage and resection of the hematoma seen in above figure. (From the NASPAG PediGYN Teaching Slide Set. Photographic image courtesy of Diane F. Merritt, M.D.)

A urethral catherter permits monitoring of urine output and gentle assessment of urethral integrity. It also protects the urethra during suturing of periurethral lacerations.

Medical Management

When surgical treatment of genital trauma is not indicated, the affected area should be cleansed two or three times per day with a solution that need not be washed away. An antiobiotic cream or ointment also can be applied sparingly. Ice packs (wrapped) may decrease swelling and provide comfort for the first 24 hours. An oral analgesic can be given, but a narcotic usually is not required. Voiding may be less painful if warm water is poured over the vulva during voiding. Exercise and activities that stretch the perineum should be avoided for about 3 to 4 weeks.

Psychological support provided with an optimistic, noncondemning attitude, rather than morose encouragement, relieves the child's guilt and long-term feelings of a terrible abnormality of her vulva. Prevention plans can be established. Follow-up in 7 to 10 days is usual, but should be sooner if the situation deteriorates.

SUMMARY

In the management of genital trauma there are three major questions that must be answered before treatment can be started. These questions are: 1) Does the child require resuscitation? 2) Is the trauma of genital origin? 3) Is the condition truly trauma or pathology masquerading as trauma? All these questions can be answered by performing a good history and a full examination. In addition, the history can be amplified by material obtained from the adult that brought the child to the emergency room. The criteria for surgical treatment, after completing the history and physical, can then be put into place. Individualization of the management of the traumatic event is dependent upon the findings, the laboratory data, and the answer to the three questions posed.

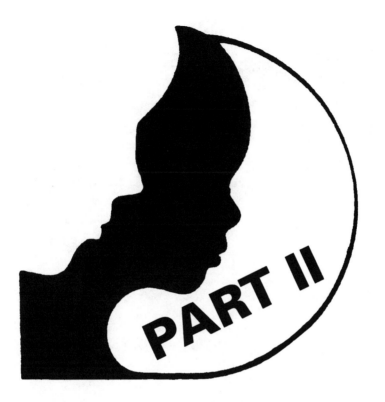

PART II

NORMAL PUBERTAL DEVELOPMENT

Peter A. Lee, M.D., Ph.D.

INTRODUCTION

Puberty is the period of attainment of adult sexual and reproductive characteristics. The development of these characteristics result from and occur concomitantly with the final changes in the maturational process of the hypothalamic-pituitary-gonadal (HPG) axis. Skeletal age (bone age) x-rays are a reflection of the biologic maturity of an individual. Pubertal events correlate with skeletal age, sometimes more closely than with chronologic age. The onset of puberty occurs in normal, healthy girls when skeletal age approximates 11 years, regardless of their chronologic age.

The events of puberty occur in an orderly sequence within a defined period of time; not only is the onset of changes expected to occur within a fairly fixed time frame but also their progression and completion can be expected to be accomplished by a defined age range. In addition to the development of sexual characteristics, gender-related somatic characteristics (e.g., alterations in lean body mass and fat distribution) occur during puberty. The final rapid period of skeletal maturation, resulting in epiphyseal fusion and adult height at the completion of growth, also occurs during puberty.

Two distinct and separate phenomena occur at the onset of puberty—adrenarche and gonadarche. *Gonadarche,* the onset of pubertal gonadal activity, is the major event; it results from HPG pubertal maturation with an upsurge of episodic gonadotropin, particularly luteinizing hormone (LH), secretion. *Adrenarche,* a relatively minor change in terms of physiologic effects, is an increase in adrenal androgen secretion that generally precedes gonadarche and occurs independently thereof. The onset of puberty is not related to body fat mass or distribution, although conversely body fat distribution is related to hormone levels during early puberty. Hormone levels in early puberty predict the rate of progression of puberty.

HYPOTHALAMIC-PITUITARY-GONADAL (HPG) AXIS

Although the triggering mechanism for the onset of puberty is not known, the hormonal changes that lead to pubertal development have been well described. It is clear that the primary driving mechanism emanates from the central nervous system, expressed by the episodic release of gonadotropin-releasing hormone (GnRH). GnRH-secreting neurons are principally located in the mediobasal hypothalamus after migration during fetal life from the olfactory bulbs. Their axons form neurovascular junctions in the median eminence. GnRH is secreted from a prohormone that is cleaved into GAP (GnRH-associated peptide) and GnRH. GnRH release is inhibited by corticotropin-releasing factor, oxytocin, and opioid peptides. Stimulation of GnRH release resides with the "GnRH pulse generator," which in fact appears to be composed of the communicating network of GnRH-secreting cells.

GnRH, in turn, binds a specific glycoprotein receptor on the pituitary gonadotropin-secreting cells, thereby stimulating release of the gonadotropins, luteinizing hormone (LH) and follicle-stimulating hormone (FSH). LH and FSH are secreted in episodic bursts, reflecting the episodic secretion of GnRH; this pattern is obligatory for the normal physiologic responsiveness of the pituitary. The GnRH drive and feedback control of the hypothalamic-pituitary-gonadal mechanism first becomes operative during fetal life. It is functional during early infancy but becomes quiescent during the years of childhood, then is reactivated with the onset of puberty. Neither the cause of the down-regulation during childhood nor the stimulus for the reactivation at puberty is well understood, although both lie within the CNS and are influenced by various neurotransmitters.

Gonadarche

At the onset of puberty (which precedes any physical changes of puberty), the irregular, low-amplitude hormonal secretion pulses characteristic of childhood become more regular, and their amplitude increases greatly. This episodic secretion first becomes apparent for LH during sleep. Before puberty, FSH levels among girls are relatively greater than LH levels and than among boys. During puberty, the magnitude and the episodic release of LH is more dramatic for LH than FSH. This maturational pattern occurs among agonadal individuals, evidence that it occurs without the requirement of gonadal feedback. The mean gonadotropin levels rise progressively until menarche.

The episodic release gradually becomes characteristic of the 24-hour day; regular daytime pulses are first seen in girls at the time of the onset of breast development. The frequency of these pulses depends upon the hormonal milieu, and is primarily influenced by estrogen and progesterone in girls. The number of pulses varies from 12 to 18 per 24-hour day; that is, they occur on the average every 90 to 120 minutes. To verify that puberty is occurring, frequent sampling to ascertain episodic release is seldom necessary. Exogenous GnRH stimulation testing stimulates a characteristic release pattern of LH and FSH, indicative of the up-regulation of the pituitary gonadotropes of puberty (Figure 5-1). Therefore, such testing is the best diagnostic tool to verify pubertal gonadotropin secretion.

Gonadotropins stimulate the secretion of estradiol and the maturation of follicles within the ovaries (LH stimulates the production of androstenedione in the theca cells

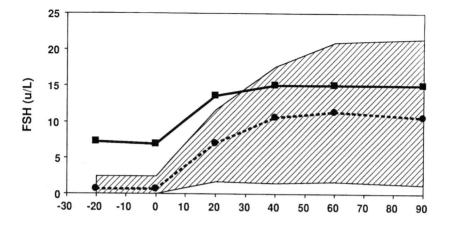

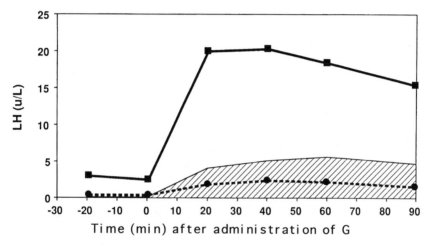

Time (min) after administration of G

Figure 5-1. GnRH stimulation testing to ascertain pubertal status of two patients. The horizontal axis is the time after administration of GnRH. The shaded area represents the normal prepubertal responses for LH and FSH in females. The patient represented by the squares and solid lines had a pubertal response (LH response above the prepubertal range and a LH:FSH ratio >1). The patient represented by the circles and dashed lines had possible early physical changes of puberty but a prepubertal response (LH response within the prepubertal range and LH:FSH ratio <1). Note that prepubertal and pubertal FSH responses tend to overlap.

of the ovary, and FSH stimulates its conversion to estradiol in the granulosa cells.) The ovaries, in turn, secrete estrogen, inhibin, perhaps follistatin, and, after ovulation, progesterone; these hormones provide negative feedback to the hypothalamus and pituitary. This onset of pubertal gonadal activities is referred to as gonadarche. Over time, after recruitment of a primary follicle and its capacity for marked estradiol secretion, the potential for positive feedback with midcycle release of gonadotropins is realized and ovulation occurs.

TABLE 5-1.   Tanner Staging of Pubertal Development in Girls

Stage Breast	Pubic Hair	Concomitant Changes
1 Prepubertal, papilla elevation	No pigmented hair	
2 Budding, larger areolae, palpable and visible elevated contour	Pigmented hair, mainly labial	Accelerated growth rate
3 Enlargement of the breast and areola	Coarser, spread of pigmented hair over mons	Peak growth rate, thicker vaginal mucosa, axillary hair
4 Secondary mound of areola and papilla	Adult type but smaller area	Menarche (stage 3 or 4), decelerated growth rate
5 Mature	Adult distribution	

Adrenarche

Preceding gonadarche, the adrenal cortex begins to secrete increased amounts of adrenal androgens. This rise, called *adrenarche,* occurs independent of gonadotropin stimulation and ovarian activity. Increased secretion of adrenal androgens is the first recognizable hormonal change of puberty. Elevation of dehydroepiandrosterone (DHEA) sulfate levels occurs first, followed by elevation of DHEA and androstenedione. Serum levels of any of these hormones can be used as hormonal evidence of adrenarche. Adrenal androgens, alone or with ovarian androgens, stimulate the onset of sexual hair, oily skin, and seborrhea or acne.

PHYSICAL CHANGES OF PUBERTY IN GIRLS

Breast Development

Usually *thelarche,* the onset of breast development, which occurs in response to ovarian estrogen secretion, is the initial sign of pubertal development among girls, although the onset of an increased statural growth rate may actually precede this. Sometimes actual breast development may be difficult to ascertain, especially in girls who have considerable subcutaneous tissue in the anterior chest. Clear signs of breast growth include outward protrusion on a nipple of increased diameter, tenting of the nipple and areolar area, increased diameter and pigmentation of the areolar area, or a palpable nubbin of breast tissue centered beneath the nipple and areola. Initial breast development may be unilateral and asymmetry may persist for varying periods of time.

Pubertal breast development marks the beginning of the Tanner stage 2 breast development (Table 5-1). Tanner staging of breast development, an artificial grading of a progressive growth process, provides a convenient description of development. The amount of breast tissue does not correlate with body mass or hormone levels; both genetic factors and body weight influence breast size.

The mean age at the onset of breast development is slightly before the eleventh birthday, although the normal age of onset varies from 8 to 13.5 years (Table 5-2). Rate of progression of pubertal development varies so that while attainment of Tanner stage 5 usually occurs within 3 to 4 years, it may occur as quickly as 1.5 years or require 5 to 6 years.

TABLE 5-2. Age of Onset of Events of Puberty in Girls

Event	Mean (years)	Range (years)
Stage 2 breast development	10.9	8.0–13.5
Stage 2 pubic hair	11.5	8.0–13.5
Peak growth rate (height)	11.9	10.2–15.0
Stage 3 breast development	12.2	10.0–14.5
Peak weight gain	12.4	9.5–15.5
Stage 3 pubic hair	12.4	10.4–14.5
Axillary hair	12.7	11.5–14.5
Acne	12.7	12.0–14.3
Menarche	12.8	10.0–16.0
Stage 4 breast development	13.2	11.0–15.5
Stage 4 pubic hair	13.2	11.0–15.8
Regular menstrual cycles	13.9	12.0–17.0
Stage 5 pubic hair (adult)	14.4	12.5–17.0
Stage 5 breasts (adult)	14.8	12.0–17.5

Pubic Hair Development

The appearance of the first coarse pigmented hairs in the genital region mark the onset of *pubarche,* pubertal pubic hair development (Tanner stage 2 pubic hair). (Note that Tanner staging is more definitive if breast development and pubic hair are designated separately since the two may not coincide.) The first growth of pubic hair is usually along the labia majora. Pubarche, the initial growth of pubic hair, may be stimulated by adrenal androgen secretion (adrenarche); later growth results from androgens of both adrenal and ovarian origin.

Onset of pubic hair growth most commonly occurs within 6 months after the onset of breast development but may precede it. Progression of pubic hair is generally more rapid than breast development, so that Tanner stage 5 pubic hair may be attained before Tanner stage 5 breast development (see Table 5-2). Full pubic hair maturity usually occurs within 2.5 to 3 years, although the range extends from 1.5 to 4.0 years.

Pubertal Genital Development

Pubertal genital development includes an increase in the size of the mons pubis and the labia majora due to deposition of subcutaneous fat. The labia minora grow in response to estrogen but do not accumulate fat subcutaneously. Clitoral growth is similar to growth of surrounding tissues. The vagina increases in length, and leukorrhea may occur early during puberty from desquamated epithelial cells and cervical mucus. The vaginal mucosa changes in response to estrogen stimulation. The initial change is the shift from predominantly parabasal cells to about 50% intermediate cells. The shift continues until, after considerable estrogen stimulation, the predominant cells are cornified. After menstrual cycles are established, a characteristic maturation pattern can be found at the various phases of the menstrual cycle. The initial growth of the uterus is myometrial, followed by endometrial development concomitant with other estrogen-stimulated changes. Uterine growth is more rapid just before menarche.

Menarche

Although the average girl experiences menarche 2 years after the onset of breast development, there is considerable variation. The mean age of menarche is 12.8 years, but it
may occur from 10 to 16 years of age. The onset of puberty and menarche are not parallel
events, although hormone levels in early puberty predict the rate of development, with
higher levels leading to earlier menarche. The majority of the cycles within the first 2
years after menarche are anovulatory; however ovulation may occur even before the
first menses. The percentage of females having ovulatory cycles gradually increases
with age. The amount and duration of menstrual flow and the length of the cycle may
vary considerably. Irregular cycles or long intervals between menses may occur at any
age and are often temporally related to emotional stress or environmental changes.

Changes in Body Composition and Proportions

Lean body mass begins to increase during early puberty in both sexes, peaking at
menarche for girls. Fat mass increases during the later stages of puberty in girls. Percentage of body water decreases during puberty because of the decrease in intracellular
water component. There are relatively minimal sex differences in build and proportions
before puberty. During adolescence, girls typically undergo a broadening of the hips
relative to the shoulders and waist. Upper/lower height ratios (upper segment–height
minus distance from pubic symphysis to floor or sitting height; lower segment–distance
from pubic symphysis to floor or standing height minus sitting height) are also similar
for boys and girls to about age 11 years. Thereafter, females ratios become greater,
because they have relatively shorter legs than boys.

The size and shape of the head and face change during puberty. Frontal sinuses and
brow ridges result in forward growth of the forehead. The posterior cranial base lowers.
Facial measurements change just after peak height gain during the peak weight gain
period. The facial profile becomes straighter with the nose growing downward and
forward. The chin becomes more pointed because of mandibular growth, and maxillary
and mandibular growth brings the teeth more upright. Among females, muscle strength
increases until 16 years of age.

Pubertal Growth Spurt

The adolescent growth spurt occurs relatively early among girls, concomitant with or
preceding thelarche, beginning as early as 8 years or as late as 12 years (Figure 5-2).
Peak growth rates generally occur during Tanner stage 2 breast development (see Tables
5-1 and 5-2). Among the sex steroids, estrogen is the most potent stimulator of somatic
growth and skeletal maturation. This is reflected in the early onset of the pubertal
growth spurt in girls and in their brisk statural growth and osseous maturation, leading
to rapid epiphyseal fusion and hence relatively less height increase during puberty
among girls than boys.

Peak height gain, which usually occurs at about 12 years of age in girls, precedes
peak weight gain. Mean maximal growth rate is 8.5 cm/y, although it may be as much
as 10.5 cm/y. Maximal weight gain occurs about 6 months later (mean age, 12.5 years)
with a rate ranging from 5.5 to 10.5 kg/y (mean, 8.5 kg/y). After menarche, additional

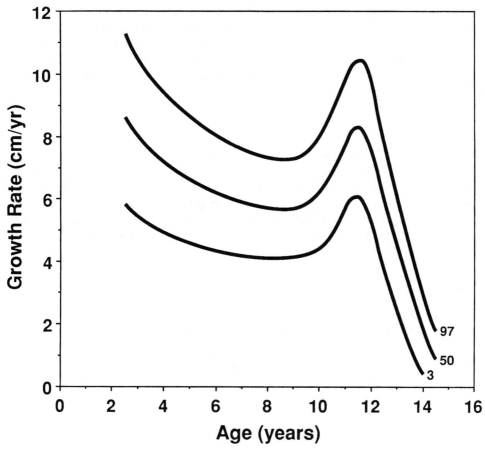

Figure 5-2. Growth rate versus age among girls. Note the pubertal growth spurt and variation thereof. If the growth rate occurs earlier or later than average, the peak rate is lower. 97, 50, 3 indicate percentiles of normal population.

growth may range from 1 to 10 cm. The often-quoted rule of 2 inches (5 cm) of growth after menarche is an average and is generally not applicable to individuals.

HORMONAL CHANGES DURING PUBERTY

Hormonal levels during each of the Tanner stages are summarized in Table 5-3.

Gonadotropins

LH and FSH are secreted by the same pituitary gonadotrope cell, although their synthesis is controlled by separate genes. During the peripubertal period before physical evidence of pubertal development, release of LH increases in response to exogenous GnRH stimulation. This increase occurs concomitantly with the sleep-related accentuation of episodic LH release. Mean circulating levels of gonadotropins gradually increase during puberty until menarche. Because of heterogeneity of the carbohydrate moieties attached to the peptide portion of gonadotropins, these hormones exist in a variety of isoforms. Biologically active LH increases in early puberty; blood levels correlate with the secretion of the more-basic isoforms.

Estrogens

Estradiol, the principal ovarian estrogen, is secreted in a fluctuating pattern in response to both LH and FSH stimulation of the granulosa and luteal cells. Mean estradiol levels increase steadily during puberty until ovulatory cycles are established. After menarche, plasma estradiol levels reach about 50 pg/ml during the early and mid follicular phase, and approximate 150 pg/ml in the late follicular phase. Estrone levels rise until mid-puberty; it is produced by conversion of estradiol and androstenedione, the latter of ovarian and adrenal origin.

Progesterone

Progesterone is an intermediate metabolite in production of the sex steroids and the principal metabolite of the corpus luteum. Levels rise minimally during puberty as steroid production is increased; after menarche progesterone levels are very high during the luteal phase of the menstrual cycle. Plasma levels of progesterone may be used as documentation of ovulation and corpus luteum formation; samples usually are obtained within 2 weeks of the date that the next menses is expected.

Androgens

Since metabolic pathway for synthesis of the sex steroids is the same in the adrenal cortex, ovaries, and testes and since several androgens are intermediate metabolites in the synthesis of estrogens, low levels of circulating androgens are part of normal female physiology. Circulating levels of dehydroepiandrosterone (DHEA) and DHEA sulfate increase progressively from 6 years of age at adrenarche throughout puberty. DHEA is of both adrenal and ovarian source, whereas DHEA sulfate is adrenal in origin. Because of the prolonged half-life of DHEA sulfate, levels of this androgen are relatively constant and tend to be a better index of adrenarche than DHEA. Androstenedione and testosterone are produced the ovaries and adrenal glands or by peripheral conversion of their precursors. Both increase slowly during pubertal development to adult female levels.

Inhibin

Inhibin, a glycoprotein, occurs in two forms that have different beta subunits. Inhibin and a related hormone, follistatin, suppress FSH secretion, while activin stimulates FSH secretion. FSH, in turn, stimulates inhibin production. Inhibin is secreted by the granulosa cells of the ovary. Its negative feedback effect, which decreases production and secretion of pituitary FSH, plays an important role during the development of the ovarian follicle as granulosa cells divide. Currently, assays for inhibin are being

TABLE 5-3. Plasma Hormone Levels (Mean and Range) during Tanner Stages of Puberty*

Hormone	(Prepubertal) Stage 1	Stage 2	Stage 3	Stage 4	Stage 5 (Adult) Follicular Phase	Luteal Phase
LH-RIA (mIU/ml)	2.7 (1–5.5)	4.2 (1–9)	6.7 (1–14.5)	7.7 (2.8–15)	7.6 (3–18)	6.6 (3–18)
ICMA (mIU/ml)	0.06 (0.02–01.8)	0.72 (0.02–4.7)	2.3 (0.1–12)	3.3 (0.4–11.7)	4.5 (2–9)	5.4 (2–11)
FIA (μ/L)	<0.1 (<0.1–0.2)	1.1 (<0.1–4.1)	2.5 (0.1–8.9)	3.2 (0.7–9.0)	3.8 (1.6–8.1)	3.5 (1.5–8.0)
FSH-RIA (mIU/ml)	4 (1–5)	4.5 (1–7.2)	6.8 (3.3–10.5)	7.4 (3.3–10.5)	10.3 (6–15)	6.0 (3.4–8.6)
ICMA (mIU/ml)	2 (1–4)	4 (1–11)	5 (1.5–13)	6.5 (1.5–13)	6.8 (1.8–13)	6.0 (1.7–12)
FIA (μ/L)	1.5 (.5–3)	2.5 (.5–3.7)	3 (1.3–4.0)	3.5 (2.8–4.5)	4.1 (2.1–7.8)	3.4 (1.8–7.6)
Estradiol (pg/ml)	9 (5–20)	15 (9–30)	27 (9–60)	55 (16–85)	50 (30–100)	130 (70–300)
Progesterone (ng/dl)	22 (7–32)	30 (10–51)	36 (10–75)	175 (10–2500)	35 (13–75)	750 (200–2500)
DHEA sulfate (μg/dl)	49 (20–95)	129 (60–240)	155 (85–290)	195 (106–320)	220 (118–320)	
After adrenarche	106 (40–200)					
DHEA (ng/dl)	35 (15–130)	300 (150–540)	328 (190–620)	395 (240–768)	540 (215–855)	
After adrenarche	130 (70–180)					
Androstenedione (ng/dl)	25 (8–50)	77 (40–112)	126 (55–190)	147 (70–245)	172 (74–284)	
Testosterone (ng/dl)	5 (3–10)	18 (7–29)	26 (10–40)	33 (16–62)	36 (21–65)	
Inhibin (not clinically available)						
SHGB (μg/dl)	3.2 (1.8–5.5)	—	1.8 (0.9–3.2)	—	2.3 (1.0–3.0)	
Prolactin (ng/ml)	(2–12)				(2.2–19.2)	
Growth hormone	Unstimulated values not useful for diagnostic purposes					
IGF₁ (ng/ml)	255 (90–420)	410 (242–578)	492 (132–850)	505 (195–815)	460 (234–686)	

*Stages based on combined breast development and pubic hair staging. Values represent a composite from the author's laboratory and normal ranges provided by commercial laboratories including Endocrine Sciences, Calabasas Hills, California.

developed. Measurements of inhibin are used primarily for research studies, and available data have little clinical usefulness in female pubertal development.

Sex-Hormone–binding Globulin (SHBG)

SHBG is a glycoprotein that binds about 99% of circulating estradiol. Only the unbound steroid is physiologically active. Levels of SHBG, which are similar in boys and girls before puberty, decrease during puberty. Plasma SHBG levels in adult men are about half those in adult women. SHBG levels are not used in assessing female pubertal development except when androgen excess is suspected; in this situation, direct or indirect (e.g., free testosterone) measurement of binding globulin may be helpful.

Prolactin

Unlike secretion of other pituitary hormones, secretion of prolactin is not stimulated by any known hypothalmic prolactin-releasing hormone. Rather, major control of prolactin secretion appears to be exhibited by a hypothalmic prolactin-inhibiting hormone. Elevated prolactin levels, indicative of defective inhibiting hormone secretion, may be an index of general hypothalamic dysfunction. Prolactin levels in girls increase somewhat during puberty, apparently largely because of stimulating effects of estrogen.

Growth Hormone (GH)

Growth hormone secretion increases during puberty, apparently because of the stimulating effects of increased sex hormones. Growth hormone, like other peptide hormones, is secreted in episodic bursts; increased GH secretion during puberty is due largely to the greater amplitude of GH secretory pulses, although the frequency of pulses also increases. The pubertal growth spurt apparently results from the increased secretion of sex steroids, particularly estradiol in girls. Sex steroids may accelerate growth by stimulating secretion of growth hormone. Generally, GH secretion is clinically useful only for evaluating deficiency. For such purposes, basal levels are seldom useful, and stimulation testing of growth hormone release is necessary.

Intrauterine Growth Factor 1 (IGF-1)

Intrauterine growth Factor 1 (IGF-1), a GH-dependent growth factor, circulates bound to proteins, particularly IGF-binding protein 3. The IGF-1 binding protein is a portion of the IGF-1 receptor; this complex regulates the action of IGF-1. Plasma levels of IGF-1 rise during early puberty, the increase being mediated by increases in GH secretion and correlated with estradiol levels. Levels remain elevated during the pubertal growth peak and then fall to adult levels. IGF-1 levels may be clinically useful as an indirect index of growth hormone status. They are not used in assessing general pubertal development, but may be useful in evaluating growth failure in adolescence.

SUMMARY

Puberty is the result of gonadarche, the pituitary gonadotropin stimulated maturation of the gonad. A minor role is also played by adrenarche, the increase of adrenal androgen production. In the usual sequence of changes, adrenarche is detectable first by an increase in circulating levels of adrenal androgens, while thelarche, the ovarian estrogen stimulated onset of breast development is the initial physical change of puberty noted. This is followed shortly by androgen stimulated pubarche, onset of sexual hair growth. Concomitantly, the pubertal growth spurt and reproductive tract growth begins. Progression of breast and pubic hair development can be tracked by Tanner staging. During mid to late puberty, menarche occurs, although the timing of the first ovulatory cycle is less predictable. Circulating hormone levels, including LH, FSH, estrogen, androgens, prolactin, and intrauterine growth factor 1, gradually rise throughout early puberty; levels after regular cycling becoming characteristic of the menstrual cycle. An marked rise of LH after GnRH stimulation testing provides an excellent index that pubertal gonadotropin secretion has begun.

SUGGESTED READINGS

Apter D, Butzow TL, Laughlin GA, et al. Gonadotropin-releasing hormone pulse generator activity during pubertal transition in girls: pulsatile and diurnal patterns of circulating gonadotropins. J Clin Endocrinol Metab. 1993;76:940.

Burger HG, McLachlan RI, Bangah M, et al. Serum inhibin concentrations rise throughout normal male and female puberty. J Clin Endocrinol Metab. 1988;67:689.

Cara JF. Growth hormone in adolescence. Endocrinol Metab Clin North Am. 1993;22:533.

deRidder CM, Thijssen JHH, Bruning PF, et al. Body fat mass, body fat distribution, and pubertal development: a longitudinal study of physical and hormonal sexual maturation of girls. J Clin Endocrinol Metab. 1992;75:442.

Forbes GB. Nutrition, growth, and development. In Sanfilippo JA (ed). *Pediatric and Adolescent Gynecology*. WB Saunders, Philadelphia, 1994; pp 128–139.

Goji K. Twenty-four hour concentration profiles of gonadotropin and estradiol (E_2) in prepubertal and early pubertal girls: the diurnal rise of E_2 is opposite the nocturnal rise of gonadotropin. J Clin Endocrinol Metab. 1993;77:1629.

Kletter GB, Padmanabban V, Brown MB, et al. Serum bioactive gonadotropins during male puberty: a longitudinal study. J Clin Endocrinol Metab. 1993;76:432.

Lee PA. Neuroendocrine maturation. In Lavery JP, Sanfilippo JS (eds). *Pediatric and Adolescent Gynecology*. Springer-Verlag, New York, 1985; pp. 12–26.

Lee PA. Pubertal neuroendocrine maturation: early differentiation and stages of development. Adolesc Pediatr Gynecol. 1988;1:3.

Lee PA. Normal ages of pubertal events among American males and females. J Adolesc Health Care. 1980;1:26.

Lee PA, Reiter EO, Kulin H. Neuroendocrinology of puberty. In Sanfilippo JA (ed). *Pediatric and Adolescent Gynecology*. Philadelphia, WB Saunders, 1994; pp 44–52.

Lee PA. Physiology of puberty. In Becker KL (ed). *Principles and Practice of Endocrinology and Metabolism*. Philadelphia, JB Lippincott, 1990; pp 740–747.

Marshall WA, Tanner JM. Variations in pattern of pubertal changes in girls. Arch Dis Child. 1969;44:291.

Martha Jr PM, Reiter EO. Pubertal growth and growth hormone secretion. Endocrinol Metab Clin North Am. 1991;20:165.

Parker LN. Adrenarche. Endocrinol Metab Clin North Am. 1991;20:71.

Rosenfield RL. Puberty and its disorders in girls. Endocrinol Metab Clin North Am. 1991;20:15.

Styne D. Normal growth and pubertal development. In Sanfilippo JA (ed). *Pediatric and Adolescent Gynecology*. Philadelphia, WB Saunders, 1994; pp 20–33.

Wheeler MD. Physical changes of puberty. Endocrinol Metab Clin North Am. 1991;20:1.

Wu FCW, Butler GE, Kelnar CJH, et al. Patterns of pulsatile luteinizing hormone and follicle-stimulating hormone secretion in prepubertal (mid childhood) boys and girls and patients with idiopathic hypogonadotropic hypogonadism (Kallmann's syndrome): a study using an ultrasensitive time-resolved immunofluorometric assay. J Clin Endocrinol Metab. 1991; 72:1229.

DYSFUNCTIONAL UTERINE BLEEDING

Alvin F. Goldfarb, M.D.

INTRODUCTION

Excess irregular uterine bleeding is a gynecologic problem for which adolescent girls may seek medical help. Excess irregular bleeding in adolescents, the subject of this chapter, is most commonly a symptom of anovulation, systemic disease, or pregnancy. Many young adolescents who use oral contraceptives develop spotting, staining, and irregular periods, which cause them to become concerned and poor compliers. (These problems are discussed in Chapter 8.) Rarely is organic disease of the uterus the cause for excess irregular uterine bleeding in the adolescent. This is in contradistinction to the mature and perimenopausal woman.

A menstrual rhythm of 21–45 days is usually established immediately following menarche. Cycles should be at the least irregularly regular even from the first menstrual period. The common belief that the anovulatory cycles of early adolescence are very irregular cannot be documented in the literature. For example, it has been stated that nearly 45% of cycles within the first year after menarche are ovulatory. Yet recent data demonstrate that the frequency of ovulation during adolescence depends largely upon the age of menarche; the earlier menarche occurs, the sooner regular ovulation is established. Apter and co-workers from Finland have stated that "the times from menarche until 50% of the cycles were ovulatory were about 1, 3, and 4.5 yr when the ages at menarche were less than 12.0, 12–12.9, and more than or equal to 13.0 yr, respectively."[1] Furthermore, their data demonstrate that it may take nearly 6–7 years after menarche before 90% or more of cycles are ovulatory.

Even though a large number of adolescent cycles are anovulatory, menstrual rhythm is maintained as described above. Following the establishment of regular ovulation, cycle length should average 29.5 days (range of 21–45 days), blood loss should average 40–100 ml per menstrual period, and the duration of flow should average 2–7 days.

MENSTRUATION: OVULATORY AND ANOVULATORY

An orderly sequence of hormonal and endometrial events is responsible for the very regular and limited bleeding that is associated with adult ovulatory cycles. Repetitive patterns of gonadotropin release are responsible for orderly follicular development and estrogen secretion during the proliferative phase of the cycle. Mid-cycle LH surges are responsible for the ovulatory process. Subsequent gonadotropin release in the luteal phase is responsible for the secretion of progesterone as well as estrogen, followed by a withdrawal of both hormones.

Estrogen stimulates the production of both estrogen and progesterone receptors on endometrial cells. Binding of estrogen to its receptors induces mRNA synthesis and subsequent production of endometrial proteins. As long as estrogen is secreted in an unopposed (i.e., without concomitant progesterone) and continuous manner, the endometrium continues to grow.

The effects of progesterone on the endometrium during the luteal phase are to halt growth and to stabilize the endometrium. Progesterone decreases the quantity of both estrogen and progesterone receptors. With fewer estrogen receptors, stimulation of the growth phase is halted. The binding of progesterone to its own receptors induces synthesis of different mRNA, which results in predecidualization of the endometrial stroma and is a very stabilizing influence. Once the corpus luteum begins its demise and estrogen and progesterone are withdrawn, an orderly sequence of hormonal (prostaglandin mediated) and vascular events occurs universally throughout the endometrium, leading to a complete sloughing and well-controlled bleeding.

Anovulation that continues pathologically into the adult years often is associated with irregular and often prolonged episodes of heavy bleeding. In these patients, progesterone either is never produced or is produced only during the infrequent ovulatory cycle. Numerous follicles are continuously being stimulated to grow by an abnormal secretion of gonadotropins (the classic LH:FSH ratio of 3:1 in polycystic ovarian disease). Increased androgen secretion (also resulting from the abnormal gonadotropin secretion) causes premature follicular atresia. The continuous unopposed secretion of estrogen from these multiple follicles of different sizes has only one effect on the endometrium: growth. The endometrium continues to grow and becomes significantly thicker than that of ovulatory cycles. It will slough after it develops to an unstable thickness or if the abnormal gonadotropin pattern is interrupted and estrogen levels drop. The latter estrogen-withdrawal menses is probably the exception. In either case, shedding of the unstable and excessively thickened endometrium is neither a universal nor orderly event. The resultant bleeding may be prolonged and uncontrolled.

Cycle lengths during adolescence do not differ appreciably from the norms of adult ovulatory cycles. Cycle lengths tend to vary more during the early menstrual years, but they stay within the range of ovulatory cycles. While most cycles during the early adolescent years are anovulatory, abnormal bleeding is rare at this time. The negative feedback system develops its own cyclicity very early. As estrogen levels rise, gonadotropin levels are suppressed. Subsequently, as gonadotropin secretion is suppressed, so is estrogen production. Endometrial shedding occurs during times of estrogen withdrawal. Menarche is usually a very limited bleeding episode because shedding occurs in the presence of an intact negative feedback mechanism and cyclic gonadotropin secretion, and at the time of an early estrogen withdrawal. This repetitive up-down relationship

Table 6-1. Etiology of Abnormal Uterine Bleeding

Pelvic Causes	Extra Pelvic Causes
• Pregnancy	• Coagulation defects
• Malignancy	• Endocrinopathies
• Infection	• Systemic diseases
• Vaginal lesions	• Medications
• Cervical lesions	
• Uterine pathology	
• Ovarian factors	

of negative feedback during the early adolescent years allows for an orderly growth of the endometrium and subsequent withdrawal bleeding before the endometrium is excessively thickened. The occasional ovulatory cycle that occurs even during the first year after menarche allows for further stabilization of this very young endometrium and on occasion more complete shedding.

Menstruation that occurs on a regular basis is usually a reflection of the physiology of the ovary and changes in the endometrium in response to the cyclic production of estradiol and progesterone. Desquamation and bleeding occur as a result of the loss or lowering of hormone production by the corpus luteum, prostaglandin secretion from the endometrial cells in association with vasospasm of the small arterioles, and necrosis of the endometrial cells. Bleeding usually is controlled by platelet plugs produced by the small blood vessels in the endometrium, prostaglandin-mediated vasoconstriction, and the slow increase in estrogen production as new follicles enter the system.

ETIOLOGY OF ABNORMAL UTERINE BLEEDING DURING ADOLESCENCE

The various pelvic and extrapelvic causes of abnormal uterine bleeding are listed in Table 6-1. It is helpful to distinguish and discuss these causes separately.

Extra Pelvic Causes

In the adolescent the extra pelvic causes of uterine bleeding include certain coagulation defects such as von Willebrand's disease (factor VIII deficiency) and platelet abnormalities that are seen in association with hypersplenism and intermittent thrombocytopenic purpura (ITP) or as an expression of leukemia. Ten percent of all adolescent females who develop any of these problems may have as their presenting symptom irregular uterine bleeding. Naturally, certain endocrine disorders may result in excess irregular bleeding or amenorrhea. These include hypothyroidism, hyperthyroidism, Addison's disease, and Cushing's disease. These endocrinopathies may present as anovulation, irregular menstrual bleeding, or premature ovarian failure (Addison's disease). In addition, excess irregular uterine bleeding may present as a sequela to various infectious diseases that affect liver function. The most common of these illnesses are the viremias such as infectious mononucleosis. In this instance, the patient may have subclinical jaundice and associated with this condition an inability to properly conjugate and

Table 6-2. Common Terms for Describing Abnormal Uterine Bleeding

- **Menorrhagia (hypermenorrhea):** cyclic excessive menstrual bleeding
- **Metrorrhagia:** bleeding (either spotting or hemorrhage) in between menstrual periods
- **Menometrorrhagia:** bleeding that is totally irregular in frequency and duration of episodes and usually is excessive
- **Polymenorrhea:** menstrual-like bleeding episodes that occur more frequently than 21 days
- **Hypomenorrhea:** Decreased amount of menstrual flow
- **Oligomenorrhea:** bleeding episodes that occur irregularly more than 40 days apart and usually in a pattern of 40 to 80 days

detoxify steroids, which are metabolized in the liver. The ingestion of any drugs (e.g., alcohol) that put stress on liver function can also cause irregular bleeding.

Pelvic Causes

Whenever a previously regular menstruating female presents with a menstrual irregularity, conception has to be considered in the differential diagnosis. Therefore, any evaluation must include a pregnancy test. There must always be concern as to whether or not the individual is having a threatened abortion, an ectopic pregnancy, a normal pregnancy, or trophoblastic disease. As a rule, malignancy of any of the pelvic organs is rather rare in adolescents. However, spotting and staining may be an associated part of an HPV (human papilloma virus) infection of the cervix (see Chapter 9). The diagnosis of HPV is usually associated with an abnormal Papanicolaou smear. Excess irregular bleeding usually is not seen with functional or organic ovarian cysts. In addition, abnormal bleeding in the adolescent may reflect endometrial infections such as tuberculous or cervical lesions (e.g., polyps or cervicitis). Finally, trauma, infections, or foreign bodies in the vagina may present with irregular bleeding.

Endometrial polyps and uterine myomas are rare in the adolescent age group. Functioning ovarian tumors, endometrosis, and ovarian lesions also are uncommon causes for irregular bleeding in adolescents. In the absence of organic pelvic causes, most excess irregular uterine bleeding seen in the adolescent population is secondary to anovulation. In most cases of anovulation, the possibility of polycystic ovarian disease must be considered. Individuals with this disease usually can be identified because much of their habitus suggests an hyperandrogenic state.

EVALUATION OF ABNORMAL UTERINE BLEEDING

History

The symptom of abnormal uterine bleeding must be evaluated by obtaining important facts that relate to the onset of the problem: (1) the immediate state of emergency; (2) past medical or family history, which may provide clues to etiology; (3) presence of known systemic or psychosocial pathology; (4) the possibility of pregnancy; (5) the nature of the abnormal bleeding; and (6) any event that preceded the onset of the symptom.

During adolescence, menorrhagia is most commonly the result of an anovulatory bleed in an individual with a deranged negative feedback system (assuming that positive feedback is yet to be developed). (See Table 6-2 for definitions of terms.) However, the

Table 6-3. Laboratory Studies for Evaluating Abnormal Uterine Bleeding

- Pregnancy test
- CBC, platelet count
- Prothrombin time (PT), partial thromboplastin time (PTT)
- Thyroid function studies
- Pelvic ultrasound
- Others as indicated

clinician must be alert for a less common but potentially more serious bleeding disorder, as well as the possibility of a pregnancy-related problem.

If cyclicity has been established within the interval range that is usual for adolescents (21–45 days) even before establishment of positive feedback, then the bleeding can be classified based on its relation to the regular withdrawal episodes. The presence of irregular heavy bleeding episodes with cycle lengths outside this usual interval range identifies patients with dysfunctional bleeding resulting from derangement of positive and/or negative feedback systems. In these cases, the potential causes of abnormal GnRH and/or gonadotropin secretion must be determined. However, psychosocial pathology, competitive athletic training, systemic disorders, and other endocrinopathies also may have an adverse effect upon the hypothalamic-pituitary unit.

Physical Examination

The general examination may be directed to identification of systemic disorders, endocrinopathies, and signs of a bleeding disorder. Hyperandrogenism may be identified by the presence of excessive hair and signs of masculinization or defeminization. Remember to look for the presence of galactorrhea. The pelvic inspection is directed towards identification of a normal or abnormal mullerian system. Duplication of the mullerian system might not be easily identified. An anterior-lateral soft vaginal mass that extends to any place along the vaginal axis is most likely an obstructed unilateral genital tract filled with old blood. Further inspection is necessary to rule out neoplasia, trauma, or the presence of foreign objects. The potential for a complication of pregnancy must be sought out.

Immediate Laboratory Evaluation

Determination of the amount of blood loss and degree of emergency is best made with CBC and differential counts. Bleeding studies should be obtained on all patients with evidence of heavy or prolonged bleeding, especially when the flow has a red coloration (Table 6-3). It is imperative to obtain not only a prothrombin time (PT) and partial thromboplastin time (PTT) but also a total platelet count, bleeding time, and clotting time. Patients with von Willebrand's disease may have normal PT and PTT studies and can be identified only based on bleeding time.

Hypothyroidism is at times a subtle diagnosis to make. All patients should have a TSH, T_4 and T_3 update done routinely with their initial evaluation.

Consideration for a further hormonal evaluation should be made at the initial blood sampling. Prior evidence of recycling failure might indicate the need to obtain blood

Table 6-4. Protocol for Evaluation and Treatment of Irregular Excessive Uterine Bleeding

History and Physical Exam
Essential Laboratory Studies

CBC and differential counts
Bleeding and clotting time
Pregnancy test
PT and PTT
TSH, T_7

Treatment of Acute Episode*

Hemoglobin <7 grams
- Consider hospitalization for further evaluation and treatment (avoid transfusion if possible).
- D&C when indicated, then progestin therapy.

Hemoglobin >7 grams
- Use progestin therapy:
  Norethindrone or norethindrone acetate 5.0 mg tid for 3 weeks *or* Estrogen 25 mg IV with norethindrone 5.0 mg bid for 3 weeks *or*

  low-dose oral contraceptive 1 tablet tid for 3 weeks

After Managing Acute Episode

- Hormonal Therapy:
  Oral contraceptives for 4 months *or* cyclically

  Medroxyprogesterone acetate (MPA), 10 mg daily for 10 days each cycle, for 4 months *or*

  Norethindrone, 10 mg daily for 10 days of each cycle, for 4 months

  Supportive iron therapy

*If no immediate improvement is obtained, consider ultrasound, endometrial sampling, or hysteroscopy. However, always try a medical approach before adopting a surgical approach.

for FSH (to rule out impending ovarian failure), LH (with FSH might identify the 3:1 ratio of polycystic ovarian disease). If the patient has signs of androgen overproduction, testosterone and DHEA sulfate levels are quick screens for ovarian and adrenal pathology, respectively. Other endocrine testing may be appropriate depending upon the level of suspicion.

TREATMENT OF ABNORMAL UTERINE BLEEDING IN ADOLESCENTS

Table 6-4 outlines a protocol for treating excess irregular uterine bleeding in adolescent patients. Hospitalization is appropriate in the following situations:

- When initial hemoglobin is < 7 g.
- When orthostatic changes are present and hemoglobin is < 10 g.
- When hemoglobin is < 10 g and bleeding is excessive.

Treatment for acute emergent bleeding may require mechanical and/or hormonal therapy. A dilatation and curettage (D&C) works for these patients because it allows for a complete emptying of the uterine cavity and a more efficient uterine contractility. Although it would be inappropriate today to immediately perform a D&C in most patients with acute emergent bleeding, it may be very helpful to begin therapy with a very thorough endometrial biopsy using a Novak curette and a 10-ml syringe. The patients who do not stop bleeding until the cavity is emptied are usually those with a bleeding disorder. This usually occurs with menarche. For those young adolescents allowing easy pelvic examinations and office biopsy a vabra aspirator may be easier to pass through the cervix than the Novak curette.

Regimens of progestins with or without estrogens is the best initial hormonal approach to these patients. Progestin compounds may be used alone in regimens over 10 days to 3 weeks if it appears that enough endometrium is remaining to allow progestin-induced stabilization. Medroxyprogesterone acetate (Provera) 10 mg may be initially given every 4 hours over 24 hours are rarely extended to 48 hours. It can then be tapered to one tablet qid × 4 days, one tablet tid × 3 days, and finally to one tablet bid × 2 weeks. This entire course of therapy extends treatment over 3 weeks and tapers slowly enough so as to avoid breakthrough bleeding. Norethindrone acetate (Norlutate) 5 mg used in the same tapering fashion may be an even better choice than Provera for those patients who have bled down to more basal levels of the endometrium. It is said that each tablet of norlutate is contaminated with 20 μcg of ethinyl estradiol. The added estrogen provides the benefit of a growth and healing effect on the endometrium (as well as increasing progesterone receptors), so that the progestin will have its maximum effect. For patients who have bled excessively and for prolonged periods of time a regimen of a combination oral contraceptive is most appropriate. Lo-ovral has been a favorite because of its potent progestin, norgestrel. Concomitant antiemetics may be necessary for any of the estrogen regimens during the initial days of high dosages.

SUMMARY

Excess irregular uterine bleeding in the adolescent must always be considered a symptom and not a disease. It most commonly is a symptom of anovulation, systemic disease, or pregnancy. This symptom must be evaluated and treated in a planned fashion. The evaluation eventually involves studies of the hematopoietic system and clotting mechanism. Thyroid function studies are always part of the evaluation. Other endocrine studies may be indicated based on the findings of the physical examination. Ancillary studies may include endometrial samplings and pelvic ultrasonography. Progestational therapy given in adequate doses will usually manage the problem. Iron therapy always is given as supportive treatment. The best method of management begins with gathering information, making a diagnosis, and then treating.

LITERATURE CITED

1. Apter D, Vihko J. Hormonal pattern of adolescent menstrual cycles. Clin Endocrinol Metab. 1983;57:82.

SUGGESTED READINGS

Apter D, Vihko J. Hormonal pattern of adolescent menstrual cycles. Clin Endocrinol Metab. 1983;57:82.

Coupey, SM, Halstrom P. Common menstrual disorders. Pediatr Clin North Am. 1989;36:551.

Kulijj, W. Adolescent menstrual disorders. In Strasburger CV (ed). *Adolescent Gynecology and Office Guide*. Baltimore, Urban and Schwarzenberg, 1990.

Kusten J, Rebar, RW. Menstrual disorders in the adolescent age group. Primary Care. 1987;14:139.

Neinstein LS. Menstrual problems in adolescents. Med Clin North Am. 1990;74:1181.

Reindollar RH. The adolescent with irregular and often heavy menses: who and when to evaluate and treat. In Cefalo RC (ed). *Clinical Decisions in Obstetrics and Gynecology*. Rockville, Md, Aspen Publishers, 1990.

Reindollar RH and McDonough PG. Adolescent menstrual disorders. Clin Obstet Gynecol. 1983.

Reindollar RH and McDonough PG. Neuroendocrine processes relevant to the childhood years. Clin Obstet Gynecol. 1987;30:63.

Southam AL, Richard RM. The prognosis for adolescents with menstrual abnormalities. Am J Obstet Gynecol. 1966;94:637.

Treolar AD, Boynton RE, Behn BG, et al. Variation of the human menstrual cycle during reproductive life. Int J Fertil. 1977;12:77.

Zacharias L, Wurtman RJ, Schatzoff M. Sexual maturation in contemporary American girls. Am J Obstet Gynecol. 1970;108:833.

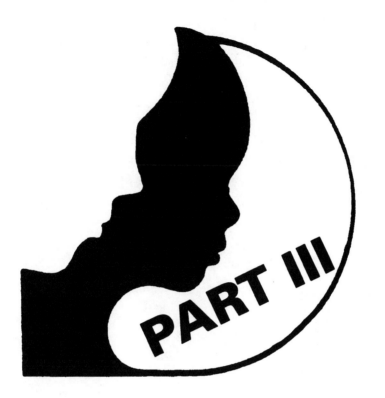

ADOLESCENT SEXUALITY

Robert T. Brown, M.D.

INTRODUCTION

Sexuality refers to much more than the behaviors intended for procreation. The term encompasses the sum of our relationships with other people, both women and men. The melding of parental gametes determines the genotypic sex of each individual; various physiological, cultural, and societal factors help to shape the phenotypic expression of that chromosomal composition. From the earliest moments of our lives the shaping begins. The answer to that first question "Is it a girl or a boy?" sets in motion a whole host of forces that direct each of us to be the kind of woman or man we will be. This discussion examines the contributions of the various factors that shape us as men and women and explores the results of that shaping in terms of how adolescents express their sexuality.

FACTORS SHAPING HUMAN SEXUALITY

Human sexuality encompasses the physical characteristics and capacities for specific sex behaviors, together with psychosocial values, norms, attitudes, and learning about these behaviors. It also includes a sense of gender identity and related concepts, behaviors, and attitudes about the self and others as men or women in the context of one's society. Although biological factors such as genotype and hormonal influences on the developing brain begin shaping sexuality from the moment of conception, the other, extrinsic, factors begin to exert their influences only after birth. The family's perception of maleness and femaleness, based on the norms and expectations of its cultures and of society in general, is expressed to the infant from the start.

Biology

Genetics assigns to individuals their genotype and the major factors in their phenotypic expression. If a person is assigned two X chromosomes, but an enzymatic defect is present in her adrenal glands, she may be born with masculinized genitalia. The reaction of her family to this whim of nature will greatly influence this girl's self-concept as a woman. If she is not fully masculinized, she still may have severe acne and/or hirsutism which will influence her self-image. As yet undetermined influences of androgens on the fetal brain may cause a particular girl to be more "boyish" than her peers, or a combination of genetic factors may make her more adept at sports. This physical capability may make her seem more "masculine" and will influence how she is perceived by others, and, ultimately, by herself.

Family

A child's first sense that he or she is a boy or girl, and what exactly that means, is conveyed by its parents from the earliest moments of life. A developing child witnesses how the mother behaves as a woman and how the father behaves as a man, and how they behave towards each other. These early impressions are the lessons that are taught best, and they go a long way in helping the child define what a man or woman should be. Modifications of these images come from other members of the family such as grandparents and siblings.

Absence of one of the parents or of someone who assumes a parental role can make it very difficult for the child to understand how a woman behaves with men and vice-versa. Girls test out how to behave as a woman with their fathers or another close adult male. Without that input, many girls may go "looking for Daddy," sometimes engaging in considerable risk-taking behavior toward that end. This search for a Daddy figure may lead to early sexual behavior with its deleterious consequences.

Inappropriate behavior on the part of her male authority figure may also color a young girl's view of sexuality. A girl who suffers from sexual abuse is likely to have a significantly impaired self-image and have difficulty establishing and sustaining hetero-sexual relationships throughout her life. On the other hand, a girl who is reared in a home in which her parents are caring, loving, supportive, and affectionate toward each other and in which the bounds of propriety are observed should be able to enter into a mature, giving relationship upon reaching adulthood.

Culture

A culture's attitude toward sex greatly influences the manner in which an adolescent can express her sexuality. First, the culture assigns men and women specific roles. When these gender roles are sharply delimited, the choices of how to express being a man or woman that are open to an adolescent are few. When the culture is ambiguous as to how the sexes are to behave, the adolescent has many options but little guidance. Similarly, the culture dictates the extent to which sexual feelings may be expressed. Cultures can be of four types in this regard: sexually repressive, sexually restrictive, sexually permissive, or sexually supportive. Each type of culture has a distinctive approach to the emergent sexuality of its youth.

A sexually repressive culture limits the overt expression of sexuality. Sexual play among the young is not allowed, and premarital chastity is required. Sexual behavior is associated with guilt, fear, and anger. Sexual pleasure has little value.

A sexually restrictive culture tries to limit the expression of sexuality. There is little sexual play in childhood, and premarital chastity is required of at least one of the sexes. This type of cultures typically is ambivalent about sex, and sex tends to be feared primarily for the problems that it can cause. The United States of the first 60 years of this century was fairly typical of this type of culture.

Tolerance of sexuality is characteristic of a sexually permissive culture. This culture loosely enforces formal prohibitions against expression of sexuality. Children may participate in sexual play as long as the adults don't see it overtly. Sex is considered a normal and valued part of human life, so sexual activity among adolescents and before marriage is accepted. Although somewhat common among non-European–based cultures, this approach to sexuality made a beachhead in the United States in the early 1960s and was adopted by increasing numbers of Americans for the next two to three decades. Because of the problems of AIDS, other STDs, and adolescent pregnancy, our culture is reverting back to the sexually restrictive view of sexuality.

Sexually supportive cultures have been especially common among the peoples of Oceania, who encourage the expression of sexuality. Sex is seen as indispensable for human happiness, and sexual experimentation is encouraged in the young. Customs and institutions supply sexual information and experience to young people of all ages; there is no such thing as a sexually latent period in a child's life.

Because the United States has a mix of cultures, Americans have diverse approaches toward and opinions about child and adolescent sexuality. For this reason, American youth may encounter conflict between the values of the culture within which they are raised and those of others with whom they interact. One impact of the "global village" of modern media is the blurring of the differences between many of the cultures in our country. Youth who spend a great deal of time watching television, for example, may come to question much more readily the cultural values imparted to them by their parents.

Society

The United States does not have a uniform culture throughout its society. Our melting pot is really more of a salad bowl, in which our various cultures blend into a (hopefully) harmonious whole but in which each component stays distinct. Conflict between the sexuality values with which adolescents are raised and those which they confront in American society at large are inevitable. Comfort and security with her own sexuality as it is learned in the home hopefully will enable the adolescent to negotiate the conflicting messages that she confronts as she matures.

One of the ways in which societal norms of sexual roles and behaviors are conveyed to adolescents is via the media, in particular television. Media exert a powerful influence on adolescents by exposing them to an adult world which they were formerly unaware. Many parents abdicate their responsibility to teach their children about sex and sexuality so, television, movies, and magazines are very important sources of information about "normal" behavior.

No other leisure activity is more widely pursued than television watching, especially among children. Adolescents watch less television than children, but what they do watch is heavily laden with messages about sexual roles and sexual behaviors.

DEVELOPMENT OF ADOLESCENT SEXUALITY

In the end, it is the mix of the above influences that determines how an adolescent will develop as a sexual being, both in terms of self-image and of behavior. To understand the sequence that occurs, it is necessary to understand basic adolescent development.

Adolescents develop in three primary areas: organic, cognitive, and psychosocial. Organic development (i.e., puberty) is discussed in Chapter 5. Cognitive development occurs in age-specific stages. Children begin to think in a formal operational manner (i.e., problem solving, inductive reasoning) at about the age of 12 years. Full capacity to think in this manner is not reached, however, until at least 15 or 16 years of age. Early (10–13 years old) and middle (14–16 years old) adolescents cannot be expected, therefore, to function in adult fashion most of the time. For example, these adolescents need concrete examples to understand ideas: in the medical setting, history taking must be specific and directive, and any instructions given to teenagers should be very concrete.

Psychosocial development encompasses an adolescent's ability to view himself or herself realistically and to relate to others. A convenient way of understanding this facet of development is to divide it into four tasks which adolescents must be well on the way to completing before they can be said to have entered adulthood. The four tasks are:

- the achievement of effective separation, or *independence*, from the family of origin;
- the achievement of a realistic *vocational* goal;
- the achievement of a mature level of *sexuality*; and
- the achievement of a realistic and positive *self-image*.

The rest of this discussion is limited to achievement of mature sexuality.

Early Adolescence

Early adolescents express their sexuality in ways that may be humorous to adults, but painful to the adolescents. They think about the opposite sex a great deal but don't do much with their thoughts (given appropriate adult supervision). Although they have numerous fantasies about the opposite sex and considerable interaction (especially in school), the social contact occurs primarily in situations created by and supervised by adults e.g., the 7th grade dance. This event is a classic situation for observing early adolescent sexuality behavior. While the girls form a mass in the middle of the dance floor, bouncing in time to the music, the boys—averaging a head shorter than the girls— circle around the outside and now and then dart toward the middle to "count coup." Occasionally, boys and girls dance together, but such interaction is tentative at best.

Middle Adolescence

As boys and girls grow into middle adolescence, their efforts at relating to those to whom they are romantically inclined center more on group dating and social activities.

Teenagers at this stage of development are more secure in their physical self-image and also more prone to spend time with others in their peer groups than younger adolescents. Any romantic involvement that they do have is normally with a partner who is of similar age. This relationship is characterized not by the giving nature of a mature relationship, but by more selfish motivations. Each participant is preoccupied with making the partner fulfill his or her fantasies of the ideal partner. Feelings are intense and, to the teenager involved, all encompassing. The partner, however, can never really match up to the image that the teenager has created; so, the relationship has, by adult standards, a very short life.

Late Adolescence

By late adolescence, teenagers usually have grown to the point where they can enter into more adult relationships. These relationships are characterized more by a concern for the feelings and welfare of their partners. The capacity for true intimacy has begun to develop, and the adolescents are capable of adult-type relationships. As this internal process proceeds, adolescents are subject to all the forces described previously and to the conditioning they received as children.

Homosexuality

Girls who will become lesbians or bisexual typically have ambiguous feelings during adolescence. It isn't until young adulthood that they begin to define clearly their gender preferences.

SUMMARY

The development of sexuality during adolescence is the summation of intrinsic biological factors and extrinsic factors including family relationships and attitudes as well as cultural and societal norms and expectations. If the process proceeds well, a young person will achieve adulthood with a good sense of self—as a woman or as a man—and with the capacity to form meaningful and lasting relationships.

SUGGESTED READINGS

Brown RT. Assessing adolescent development. Pediatr Ann 1978;7:16.

Currier RL. Juvenile sexuality in global perspective. In Constantine LL, Martinson FM (eds). *Children and Sex: New Findings, New Perspectives*. Boston, Little, Brown & Co., 1981; pp 9–19.

Hayes CD (ed). *Risking the Future*. Washington, DC, National Academy Press, 1987.

Remafedi G. Adolescent homosexuality: psychosocial and medical implications. Pediatrics 1987;79:331.

Strasburger VC. Normal adolescent sexuality: a physician's perspective. Semin Adolesc Med. 1985;1:101.

CHAPTER 8

GENITAL HUMAN PAPILLOMAVIRUS INFECTION IN ADOLESCENTS

Walter D. Rosenfeld, M.D.

INTRODUCTION

Genital infection with human papillomavirus (HPV) results in condylomata acuminata, flat warts, and cervical cytologic abnormalities. The presence of this infection becomes known when lesions are discovered by the patient or clinician, when specific laboratory tests are performed, or quite commonly when the Papanicolaou (Pap) smear is reported as abnormal. Furthermore, many episodes of HPV infection are completely asymptomatic and would only be discovered if sophisticated molecular tests were utilized. Although individuals with asymptomatic infections sometimes may transmit HPV to a sexual partner, generally neither the partner nor the patient will suffer any adverse health consequences. Consequently, a key consideration in planning the clinical care of a specific patient is that the mere presence of HPV and the finding of an abnormal Pap smear do not have the same significance.

The management of HPV infection in adolescents deserves special emphasis because the clinical significance of infection in this population differs in two respects from that of the same infection in adult women. First, the psychosocial aspects of health care for adolescents may impact upon the management of this problem. Factors such as inadequate understanding and insight into a truly complicated problem, too much or too little concern about the issue, apprehension about confidentiality, and body image concerns may affect compliance with appointments and therapeutic regimens. Second, the epidemiology and natural history of this sexually transmitted infection is such that while the highest rates occur in adolescents and young adults, the occurrence of high-grade neoplastic lesions is relatively rare in this age group.

Table 8-1. HPV Types and Diseases Produced

HPV type	Site of infection/disease
1,4	Plantar warts
2	Common warts on hands
3, 10, 28	Juvenile flat warts on arms (verrucae planae)
5, 8, 9, 12, 19–25, 36, 40	Epidermodysplasia verruciformis, with frequent progression to skin cancer
7	Common warts of meat and animal handlers
13, 32	Oral focal epithelial hyperplasia (Heck's disease), with possible progression to carcinoma
26–29, 34	Common and flat warts in immunosuppressed; nongenital Bowen's disease
6, 11, 42	Anogenital condyloma acuminatum; low-grade squamous intraepithelial lesion (LSIL) of the cervix; laryngeal papillomas
16, 18, 31, 33, 35, 39, 41–45, 51–56	Anogenital condyloma acuminatum; high-grade squamous intraepithelial lesion (HSIL) of the cervix; anogenital tract cancers

SIGNIFICANCE OF HPV INFECTION

Although much is still unknown about the biology and natural history of HPV infection, there is no doubt that HPV is closely linked with cervical neoplastic disease. In fact, it is likely that this virus is etiologically involved in the vast majority of cervical cancers, as 80%–95% of these cancers are found to contain HPV DNA. A number of characteristics of HPV have an impact upon diagnosis and management of infection. The most prominent problems include the following:

- HPV cannot be propagated in tissue culture.
- Antibodies specific for HPV have not as yet been identified, making serologic testing impossible.
- The incubation period is extremely variable, ranging from 1 to 20 months or more.
- The site of infection, as well as the specific disease produced, are dependent on the HPV type involved (Table 8-1).

Recognition of HPV infection as a sexually transmitted disease (STD), including its value as a possible indicator of sexual abuse in children, its link with cervical cytological abnormalities, and its etiologic association with other diseases (e.g., laryngeal papillomatosis, Bowen's disease, epidermodysplasia verruciformis), have prompted much recent interest. However, its link with cervical cancer is the area undergoing greatest scrutiny.

EPIDEMIOLOGY

Epidemiologic evidence implicating a sexually transmitted pathogen as a causative cofactor in cervical cancer has been recognized for some time. Supportive evidence includes the well-known positive association between number of sexual partners and risk for this cancer. Also, women with a high-risk male partner are at greater risk. That is, a woman whose male sexual partner has had penile cancer or who has had a previous female partner with cervical cancer is at increased risk. Biologic evidence linking HPV and cervical cancer include the findings that papillomaviruses are oncogenic, flat condyloma of the cervix (diagnostic of HPV) are often indistinguishable from dysplasia, and, most importantly, certain HPV types are regularly present in cervical cancer tissue.

Given that HPV is believed to be etiologically related to cervical cancer and that sexually active adolescent girls have HPV prevalence rates of 50% or more, there is a discrepancy that needs to be explained. That is, why is it that so many adolescents are infected with the virus and yet relatively few women later develop cancer? One obvious factor is the existence of extensive Pap smear screening programs, which permit early intervention. Abundant evidence exists to justify the value of this screening including the fact that cervical cancer is still a leading cause of death in women from underdeveloped countries where widespread Pap smear testing does not take place. Other factors undoubtedly also influence whether or not infection with the virus results in cervical disease. These include the role of the host immune system, the presence of cocarcinogens such as cigarettes, the specific HPV type involved (e.g., HPV-16 is more likely to be associated with high-grade neoplasia than HPV-11), and other biologic properties that result in latency, regression, or persistence of infection.

DIAGNOSIS

Condyloma acuminatum, vulvar lesions, and Pap smear abnormalities are some of the manifestations of HPV infection. Diagnosis is made by visual inspection, colposcopic examination, cytologic or histologic analysis of cells or tissue from the anogenital area, immunohistochemistry studies, or nucleic acid hybridization techniques. Visual inspection is fine when lesions are exophytic and are located in a visible area not obscured by hair or folds of mucosa, but it is not helpful in other circumstances.

Colposcopic examination, especially when coupled with application of acetic acid to the site, by far surpasses the best inspection possible with the naked eye. However, this procedure has several limitations. For example, many false-positive as well as some false-negative results occur, biopsy of suspicious areas generally is necessary, and the need for expensive office equipment, as well as considerable experience and time on the part of the examiner, make this procedure costly.

An obvious prerequisite to cytologic or histologic analysis is the collection of a specimen, from a cytologic scraping, a cervicovaginal lavage, or a colposcopic-directed biopsy. Although Pap smear screening has become a regular part of medical care for women and is clearly a life-saving procedure, important limitations in regard to its sensitivity, specificity, and quality control have been described. Histologic analysis remains the gold standard by which definitive diagnosis and treatment is based. This, of course, requires a tissue specimen, most often obtained by biopsy after an initial cytologic sample has been found to be abnormal.

Several techniques can be used to identify specific nucleic acid sequences using known HPV DNA probes. Such molecular testing not only permits accurate diagnose of infection, but also identification of the specific HPV type involved. The *dot blot* test commercially available (e.g., ViraPap/ViraType, Life Technologies, Inc, Gaithersburg, Maryland) requires collection of an additional specimen during a pelvic examination; this specimen is placed in a collection tube and then sent to a laboratory for analysis.

Table 8-2.   Treatment of Condylomata

Nonsurgical options	Surgical options
• Podophyllin	• Excision
• Trichloracetic acid	• Cryosurgery
• 5-FU	• Electrocauterization
• Interferon	• Laser
• Podofilox (Condylox®)	• Loop electrosurgical excision procedure (LEEP)

In situ hybridization is used to identify segments of HPV DNA within histologic speci- mens or within individual cells. Of greater sensitivity and specificity than these two techniques is the *Southern blot* test. Purified DNA extracted from a specimen is digested with restriction enzymes, put through an agarose gel for electrophoresis, and then transferred onto a nitrocellulose membrane. The membrane then is washed with a buffer containing radiolabeled DNA probes, which bind only to complementary DNA sequences, and an autoradiogram is produced. The bands produced on the film indicate a positive signal and allow the identification of specific HPV types.

Polymerase chain reaction (PCR) is not actually a means of identification but is an amplification technique whereby millions of copies can be made from a single HPV genome. The products of this amplification are then identified utilizing dot blot, South- ern blot, or another identification method. The extreme sensitivity of PCR makes this technique quite valuable but increases the risk of false-positive test results; thus PCR is limited to only the more sophisticated laboratories. RNA probes are used in a relative new methodology called **hybrid capture** which permits the amount of HPV DNA present to be quantified. To date this technique has been used only for research purposes.

MANAGEMENT OF HPV PATIENTS

Treatment of Condylomata

A number of options are available for treatment of condylomata, some of which may also be used when attempting to eradicate histopathologic lesions (Table 8-2). Topical application of podophyllin or trichloracetic acid is often effective and probably the treatment used most routinely. Podofilox (Condylox®, Oclassen Pharmaceuticals, Inc., San Rafael, California), a derivative of podophyllin, offers the advantage that the patient can self-treat herself after an initial office visit. Much optimism accompanied the initial use of intralesional interferon and some of the surgical modalities, but the reality is that no therapy is even near 100% effective and all are associated with some risks and morbidity. Factors complicating treatment include resistance of the virus to the specific method chosen, high prevalence rates of HPV resulting in repeated new exposures to the virus, and presence of viral DNA in sites contiguous to the area of treatment.

Role of Cytologic and Histologic Findings

Cytologic diagnosis is currently the most important method used to guide initial man- agement of cervical disease since neoplasia is the most serious consequence of HPV infection. However, it must be kept in mind that Pap smears should be used for screening and not for making a definitive, specific diagnosis. Depending upon the adequacy of

Table 8-3. Cervical Cytologic Diagnoses Most Relevant to Adolescents. (Adapted from 1991 Bethesda System of Classification)

A. Benign cellular changes
   1. Infection
      - *Trichomonas vaginalis*
      - Fungal organisms
      - Predominance of coccobacilli consistent with shift in vaginal flora
      - Bacteria morphologically consistent with *Actinomyces* spp.
      - Cellular changes associated with herpes simplex virus
      - Other
   2. Reactive changes consistent with:
      - Inflammation
      - Atrophy
      - Radiation
      - Intrauterine device
      - Other
B. Epithelial cell abnormalities
   1. Squamous cell
      a. Atypical squamous cells of undetermined significance (ASCUS). (Should be further qualified, if possible, as to whether a reactive or neoplastic process is favored.)
      b. Low-grade squamous intraepithelial lesion (LSIL) encompassing:
         - cellular changes associated with HPV (previously termed koilocytosis, koilocytotic atypia, and condylomatous atypia)
         - mild dysplasia/cervical intraepithelial neoplasia grade 1 (CIN 1)
      c. High-grade squamous intraepithelial lesion (HSIL) encompassing:
         - moderate dysplasia/CIN 2
         - severe dysplasia/carcinoma in situ/CIN 3
      d. Squamous cell carcinoma

the specimen, cytopathologic interpretation, and the patient's characteristics, follow-up will entail anything from observation and repeat sampling, to colposcopy with biopsy, to a more extensive histologic analysis using loop electrosurgical excision procedure (LEEP). The Bethesda system of classification, developed in 1988 and modified in 1991, has now become the most widely accepted standard for classification of Pap smears. As Pap smear results are not always diagnostic and are subject to more than one interpretation, the Bethesda system by its descriptive nature is intended to encourage communication between cytopathologists and clinicians. In addition to defining cytologic changes, the report should comment on the adequacy of the specimen and whether or not endocervical cells are present. The categories most relevant to adolescents include descriptions of infection, (e.g., *Trichomonas vaginalis*) and of squamous cell abnormalities (Table 8-3).

Atypical Squamous Cells of Undetermined Significance (ASCUS)

The mildest and least specific squamous cell abnormality described is atypical squamous cells of undetermined significance (ASCUS). Here the cytopathologist is encouraged whenever possible to indicate whether reactive changes are present, perhaps in association with severe inflammation, or if a neoplastic process is favored. When ASCUS is found in association with reactive changes, especially if infection with STDs such as chlamydia or trichomoniasis are known or suspected, then the patient should be given specific treatment for the infection and have a repeat Pap smear in 2 to 3 months. If the diagnosis of ASCUS is qualified by a statement favoring a low-grade squamous intraepithelial lesion (LSIL), then the approach should closely conform to the one suggested when LSIL is definitively identified (see next section). Of course, other factors need to be considered in the management plan such as the degree of risk for the patient. For example, if an adolescent has a record of poor follow-up compliance or has had previous abnormal Pap smears, colposcopy should be considered.

Low-Grade Squamous Intraepithelial Lesion (LSIL)

Underlying the approach to management of low-grade squamous intraepithelial lesions are several competing factors. First, the majority of cases with LSIL will revert to normal without any treatment whatsoever. Second, as mentioned already, the Pap smear is intended as a screening test. Some patients with LSIL on cytologic examination will actually be found to have more advanced neoplastic lesions when a more thorough evaluation is performed on a specimen obtained by biopsy. And last, even when the diagnosis of LSIL is confirmed by histologic analysis, there is currently no way to sort out the few women (albeit a very small minority of the total with LSIL) who will have progression to malignant lesions.

A number of strategies are considered acceptable in the management of a patient found to have LSIL on Pap smear. When the necessary resources are available, colposcopic examination with endocervical curettage and biopsy of any areas that appear abnormal is the approach most often utilized. Repeating Pap tests every 4 to 6 months is also considered an acceptable approach when compliance with repeat visits seems likely. However, when colposcopy is possible and practical, the procedure usually is undertaken, especially with adolescents who may not fully comprehend the importance of repeat testing.

Use of screening techniques such as HPV DNA typing and cervicography have been the subject of much debate. Although these methodologies would seem to have the capability of identifying patients at greater risk, there are some serious limitations in their sensitivity and specificity. Spurious results are likely to lead either to the performance of other tests or procedures that are unnecessary or to misguided reassurance of a patient who may still be at risk. These concerns coupled with the added costs involved with the procedures has led to recommendation that these ancillary techniques be used selectively by clinicians who have a clear understanding of their limitations.

When LSIL is histologically confirmed, a number of therapeutic options are to be considered. Laser, cryosurgery, or another procedure may be used to excise or ablate a fully visualized lesion. Following this, the patient should have repeat colposcopic examinations and Pap tests performed every 4 to 6 months until these are consistently normal. Observation plus repeat Pap tests is an option even when it is not possible to visualize the entire lesion or the limits of the transformation zone. Cervical conization in adolescent patients should probably be reserved for those who are not likely to return for follow-up, who have a higher than usual risk for malignancy, (e.g., young women who are immunocompromised due to HIV infection, transplant recipients on immunosuppressive therapy, etc.), or who have had high-grade SIL lesions in the past. Eradication of a lesion might seem to be the only appropriate option when a precancerous condition is known to exist: however, the recommendation to observe with repeat testing is based on the finding that 60% of patients with LSIL will undergo spontaneous regression. Of course in making decisions about treatment options, the risks of both the disease and the procedure need to be considered and discussed with the patient and, if possible, her parents.

High-Grade Squamous Intraepithelial Lesion (HSIL)

High-grade squamous intraepithelial lesion (HSIL) found on cytological tests should always be followed-up with colposcopy and directed biopsy. It should be emphasized that even though HSIL and invasive cancer are still uncommon in adolescents, they do occur. Definitive treatment will depend on the extent and grade of the lesion, its location, and the resources available. Loop electrosurgical excision procedure (LEEP) is now widely used, but this can produce a thermal artifact, compromise pathological examination, and may not be appropriate when the limits of the lesion or the transformation zone are not fully visible.

Counseling Issues

One of the thorniest aspects in the management of HPV infection is the need to effectively communicate information to patients about the relevant issues. Because much is still unknown about the topic, there is ongoing debate among researchers and clinicians concerning the ideal diagnostic and management strategies. The sense that one is dealing with a "descent into papillomavirus hell," as one author stated, is a sentiment often heard from involved clinicians.

Difficulties in counseling HPV patients arise in part because the relevant concepts are complicated and often seem to be contradictory. For example, the presence of genital warts is a visible and concrete expression of HPV infection, but this is usually the clinically less significant manifestation of infection when the same patient has an HPV-related abnormality on her Pap smear. Furthermore, cervical cytologic abnormalities caused by HPV (a laboratory finding) more often than not occur in women who previously have not had any other manifestations of infection. The variable and sometimes long incubation period makes determination of when infection occurred and from whom it was acquired often impossible to ascertain. There are a number of important concepts that when explained carefully can be reassuring to the patient and may enhance her trust in the clinician, thereby improving the possibility for adherence to the therapeutic regimen. It is reasonable to admit that all of the answers are not known concerning the significance of infection with HPV. On the other hand, delivery of a clear and positive approach to management is essential.

The initial task is to define the problem and explain treatment options and possible outcomes in a manner that promotes the appropriate level of concern while helping the patient to maintain a reasonable perspective on her condition. This is difficult enough with adult patients; it can be near impossible with adolescents, who commonly believes that they are immune from any danger. This frustrating, but normal adolescent attitude is encountered by clinicians on a regular basis. Use of scare tactics or exaggeration of the facts in response to this adolescent thinking is most often ineffective and counterproductive.

A better approach with a typical HPV-infected young woman is to explain that even though most patients with her type of "low-grade" abnormality undergo spontaneous resolution, there is no way to know whether or not she has a more advanced lesion without performing colposcopy. Furthermore, to make sure that she is not in the small minority of patients destined to progress from a low-grade to high-grade lesion, she will need to have repeat colposcopy and Pap smear examinations with some frequency. From the teenager's perspective compliance means that she needs to undergo a procedure that will disrupt her daily routine multiple times, may be somewhat painful, and in addition could cause difficulties in maintaining confidentiality if she does not want her parents to know about the problem. How does one convince such a young person to comply with the suggested management plan?

Compliance is most likely when information is presented at a developmentally appropriate level and in a straightforward manner. Rather than delivering a lecture on the topic, the clinician should engage the patient in a give-and-take discussion, while carefully observing both verbal and nonverbal cues. This counseling style also gives the clinician the opportunity to address concerns, misconceptions, and unanticipated anxieties most relevant to each young person. For example, the coincidental similarity between HPV and HIV, the abbreviation for human immunodeficiency virus, results in much anxiety for adolescent patients. It is often only when the clinician states (even without a query from the patient) that "HPV is a completely different virus from HIV, is not associated with AIDS, and does not cause any of the same problems" that the facial muscles of the patient relax and she smiles, a telltale sign that she was too afraid to ask a question on the subject.

Because HPV is a sexually transmitted infection, the patient may feel the stigma that often accompanies diagnosis of any STD. Most patients are reassured to learn that because HPV is so highly prevalent, variably persistent, and is most often asymptomatic, a person does not have to have had a dozen sexual partners to become infected. It can even be stated with some certainty that among sexually active young people who have had more than one lifetime sexual partner or whose partner has had other sexual contacts, the infection is probably near-ubiquitous. Furthermore, the majority of youth (including males) who have had HPV infection, whether or not they are not aware of it, are unlikely to suffer any adverse health consequence.

The Male Partner of HPV-Infected Females

The question of how to manage male partners of females with abnormal Pap test results or other manifestations of HPV is raised quite regularly. There is little evidence to date that applying aggressive diagnostic and therapeutic regimens to males with condyloma acuminatum or flat condyloma (visible with magnification after application of acetic acid) makes a significant difference in the potential for transmission to, or progression, of HPV disease in that patient's female partner. The other point to be considered is that the use of invasive tests such as urethroscopy and cystoscopy may result in retrograde infection of more proximal areas of the urethra and bladder. This could be too great a price to pay in a male who is asymptomatic, especially when the benefits to his partner are dubious.

Nonetheless, an office visit with the male partner of an infected female is indicated and often very useful. Condylomata, if present, can be identified and treated. The visit also provides an opportunity to discuss the significance of HPV, to discuss prevention of STDs, and to screen for STDs including HIV when appropriate, as well as to review pregnancy prevention and regular use of condoms.

The current medical literature is exceedingly clear that adolescents with Pap tests demonstrating ASCUS or LSIL and those with other HPV lesions (e.g., condyloma acuminatum) should at a minimum have Pap tests repeated more frequently than is generally recommended. This might be every 3, 4, or 6 months depending on the circumstances. Thus the most important aspect of managing adolescent girls with HPV infection is insuring that follow-up cervical cytologic examinations for prevention of malignancy take place. Few teenagers will be interested in hearing the debate about whether testing for HPV DNA is efficacious. Most will want to know that the Pap test, which is easy to perform, relatively inexpensive, and widely accessible is still considered the recommended screening test for cervical neoplasia.

Normative behavior among adolescents is to have serial monogamous relationships. Clinicians should not assume that a teenager who is in a "stable" relationship and has no intention of "ever" having another sexual partner is free of risk from HPV or other STDs and HPV-related Pap smear abnormalities. All adolescent girls who have begun sexual activity, even if they are not currently sexually active, should have at least an annual pelvic examination and Pap test performed. This routine annual visit, as well as consultations for an HPV-related problem, affords the clinician the opportunity to discuss issues of prevention, and when appropriate to screen for HIV and other STDs. It also presents an important opportunity to discuss pregnancy prevention and review contraceptive needs.

SUMMARY

Human papillomavirus infection and its management in adolescents is complicated by multiple factors. The fact that infection and low-grade cervical cytological abnormalities is so common contrasted with the infrequent occurrence of high-grade neoplastic lesions, presents dilemmas for the doctor and patient alike. Whether to test for the presence of the virus using molecular methodologies, how often to screen patients, and selection of the ideal treatment modality are currently debated questions. What is clear is that HPV is associated with both low- and high-grade neoplastic lesions and that the Papanicolaou smear when performed properly and regularly is a useful means of screening for significant neoplasia. Also essential in the management of adolescents is to take the time to explain and answer questions about some of the complicated aspects of this problem in a developmentally appropriate manner. As HPV related issues will be one of the most frequently seen problems among sexually active adolescent women, visits related to this afford clinicians an opportunity to counsel patients about STD's, contraception, sexual partner involvement, and other related matters.

SUGGESTED READINGS

Broder S. Rapid communication: the Bethesda system for reporting cervical/vaginal cytologic diagnoses: report of the 1991 Bethesda Workshop. JAMA. 1992;267:1892.

Diagnostic and Therapeutic Technology Assessment (DATTA). Human papillomavirus DNA testing in the management of cervical neoplasia. JAMA. 1993;270:2975.

Galloway DA. Navigating the descent into papillomavirus hell. J Infect Dis. 1994;170:1075. Editorial.

Gutman LT. Human papillomavirus infections of the genital tract in adolescents. Adoles Med: State of the Art Reviews. 1995;6:115.

Hillard PA, Biro FM, Wildey L. Complications of cervical cryotherapy in adolescents. J Reprod Med. 1991;36:711.

Hippelainen MI, Hippelainen M, Saarikoski S, Syrjanen K. Clinical course and prognostic factors of human papillomavirus infections in men. Sexually Transmitted Dis. 1994;21:272.

Koss LG. The Papanicolaou test for cervical cancer detection: a triumph and a tragedy. JAMA. 1989;261:737.

Koutsky LA, Holmes KK, Critchlow CW, et. al. A cohort study of the risk of cervical intraepithelial neoplasia grade 2 or 3 in relation to papillomavirus infection. N Engl J Med. 1992;327:1272.

Kurman RJ, Henson DE, Herbst AL, Noller KL, Schiffman MH. The 1992 National Cancer Institute Workshop. Interim guidelines for management of abnormal cervical cytology. JAMA. 1994;271:1866.

Lungu O, Sun XW, Felix J, et al. Relationship of human papillomavirus type to grade of cervical intraepithelial neoplasia. JAMA. 192;267:2493.

National Cancer Institute Workshop. The 1988 Bethesda system for reporting cervical/vaginal cytological diagnoses. JAMA. 1989;262:931.

Rosenfeld WD, Rose E, Vermund SH, et al. Follow-up evaluation of cervicovaginal human papillomavirus infection in adolescents. J Pediatr. 1992;121:307.

ACUTE AND CHRONIC PELVIC PAIN

Karen J. Kozlowski, M.D.

INTRODUCTION

The adolescent presenting with pelvic pain is a challenge to the physician. Acute and chronic pelvic pain accounts for a substantial number of consultations to gynecologists who treat adolescents. The reasons are fairly simple: first, there is the tendency to assume that "pain below the belly button" is gynecologic in origin; and second, most physicians are reluctant to perform pelvic examinations in adolescent females and often defer this to the gynecologist.

Classically, the causes of pelvic pain are divided into acute versus chronic and gynecologic versus nongynecologic. The differences between acute and chronic may not be as distinct in the adolescent as in the mature adult. The teenager experiencing her first episode of dysmenorrhea, which is typically chronic in nature, may present acutely to the emergency room. Due to her unfamiliarity with this condition, the first episode may be interpreted as acute and severe; hence, medical attention is immediately sought.

When evaluating a patient with pelvic pain, the physician not only needs to differentiate acute versus chronic, but also must consider the differential diagnosis of pelvic pain (Table 9-1). Many nongynecologic causes of pain can masquerade or be misinterpreted as gynecologic in origin. Thorough investigation should cover the wide variety of gynecologic, nongynecologic, and functional or psychosomatic causes.

HISTORY

Given the vast array of possible causes of pelvic pain, a thorough and complete history is essential. This should be obtained confidentially. A baseline menstrual history is important, including age of menarche, regularity of menses, date of last menstrual

Table 9-1.   Differential Diagnosis of Pelvic Pain

Gynecologic Causes	**Urologic Causes**
Pregnancy	Cystitis
Intrauterine	Pyelonephritis
Ectopic	Renal calculi
Ovarian cysts	Interstitial cystitis
Ovulation (Mittelschmerz)	
Torsion	**Other Causes**
Ovarian	Orthopedic diseases
Parovarian (hydatid of Morgagni)	Lordosis
Pelvic inflammatory disease	Scoliosis
Acute	Herniation of intervertebral disc
Chronic	Myofascial pain
Pelvic adhesions	Hidden agenda
Dysmenorrhea	Substance abuse
Primary	School avoidance
Secondary	Contraception
Endometriosis	Psychosocial stress
Congenital genital tract anomalies	Psychosexual trauma (physical/sexual abuse)
Gastrointestinal Causes	Somatization
Constipation	Hernia
Irritable bowel syndrome	Inguinal
Inflammatory bowel disease	Umbilical
Crohn's disease	Incisional
Ulcerative colitis	
Appendicitis	
Gastroenteritis	
Gallbladder disease	
Intestinal obstruction	
Mesenteric adenitis	
Lactose intolerance	
Pancreatitis	

period, presence of dysmenorrhea, and if dysmenorrhea is present, the age of onset, as well as any other menstrually related or cyclic pain. A specific pain history should describe the location, frequency, and duration of the pain. What exacerbates or relieves the pain, any relationship and timing of the pain to menses, urinary tract symptoms, bowel symptoms and patterns, and associated nausea and/or vomiting should be assessed. A careful and confidential sexual history should be obtained to determine any previous sexually transmitted diseases or pelvic inflammatory disease, and current risks for sexually transmitted diseases. The extent to which the pain interferes with daily activities, school work, extracurricular activities, and social functions should be evaluated, paying close attention to the number of days of school missed secondary to the pain. Any type of previous medical therapy, both prescription and nonprescription, should be determined and the extent of relief with this therapy noted. Past medical and surgical history is important, including current medications and allergies. A psychiatric history should be elicited with key questions to assess for depression. Family history should be obtained, especially for gynecologic entities such as endometriosis and pain syndromes.

A thorough social history is invaluable. School performance should be assessed as well as relationships with parents, family, and peers. Use/abuse of tobacco, alcohol, and illicit drugs should be determined. Careful questioning will often elicit any past history of sexual and/or physical abuse. All previous diagnostic procedures and treatment trials should be recorded and previous medical records obtained.

PHYSICAL EXAMINATION

A complete physical examination should be performed, paying special attention to the abdomen and pelvis to localize the pain, define the presence of masses, and assess for peritoneal signs and for organomegaly. Special care should be taken to differentiate deep pain from abdominal wall tenderness, especially in patients who have had previous surgical procedures. A pelvic examination must be performed on every patient. Ideally, speculum exams should be done in all patients to identify any vaginal or cervical anomaly. While not always feasible in the nonsexually active patient, in sexually active patients, speculum exams must be done not only to evaluate the vaginal and cervical anatomy, but to obtain cultures, wet prep, and cytologic specimens. The bimanual examination should assess uterine size, shape, and symmetry; the presence of adnexal and/or cervical motion tenderness; and identify any adnexal mass or thickening. The posterior cul-de-sac should be assessed for pain and nodularity. The rectal exam assists in evaluating the cul-de-sac and the posterior surface of the genital tract structures, as well as the rectum for constipation and fecal blood.

OTHER DIAGNOSTIC APPROACHES

Laboratory work-up should include a complete blood count with differential; a urinalysis and, as indicated, a urine culture; a pregnancy test in the sexually active teenager; and cervical cultures in the sexually active teenager. Other hematologic and biochemical studies are ordered depending on the clinical indications.

A pelvic ultrasound is valuable to confirm the presence of a mass, provide information regarding a suspected genital tract anomaly, identify the presence of free fluid in the cul-de-sac, evaluate a pregnancy, and assess the abdomen and pelvis when a satisfactory abdominal pelvic exam is not possible. Although helpful, sonography probably is not advisable in patients in whom satisfactory examinations can be accomplished. Certainly, a negative pelvic ultrasound does not rule out all possible causes of pelvic pain. In a study done at the Cleveland Clinic, Gidwani found that of 96 adolescent patients with chronic pelvic pain who were evaluated by ultrasound, 15 had a pelvic mass detected by ultrasound but only 5 were confirmed by laparoscopy.

Other radiologic evaluations may be indicated based on the diagnostic impression after completion of the history, physical examination, and a baseline laboratory work-up. These include gastrointestinal, urologic, and orthopedic studies.

Laparoscopy is an invaluable tool in the evaluation of pelvic pain. It can diagnose the presence of a specific organic disease or confirm the presence of a suspected entity that could not be demonstrated by physical exam, lab studies, or radiologic or sonographic examinations. Laparoscopy also allows the clinician to perform the appropriate biopsies and/or cultures and to treat many disorders (e.g., ablation of endometriosis, lysis of adhesions, and aspiration or excision of ovarian cysts). The most common laparoscopic findings in adolescent females with pelvic pain include endometriosis, pelvic adhesions, chronic pelvic inflammatory disease, and ovarian cysts. Other findings include uterine malformations, pelvic congestion, hydrosalpinx, and bowel disorders. Negative laparoscopies occur in a significant percentage of females. Negative findings, and the reassurance they provide that pelvic structures are normal, often leads to symptomatic improvement in adolescent females with pelvic pain. Goldstein reported that 74% of these patients were symptomatically improved after a negative laparoscopy. Some patients with pelvic pain and negative laparoscopies will improve with adjunctive psychological therapy or with the evaluation and treatment offered by intensive pain programs.

ETIOLOGY AND TREATMENT OF PELVIC PAIN

Although it is beyond the scope of this chapter to delineate all causes of pelvic pain, the more common conditions seen in the adolescent female with pelvic pain are described here.

Pregnancy

Given the high percentage of female adolescents who are sexually active (75% by age 19), it is wise to obtain a pregnancy test on adolescent patients who present with abdominal pelvic pain. Pelvic pain can occur with a normal intrauterine pregnancy, a threatened miscarriage, or an ectopic pregnancy. In an intrauterine pregnancy, pain can be the result of round ligament syndrome due to stretching of the round ligaments; "morning sickness" with the associated nausea and abdominal pain; urinary tract infections, which are seen with increased frequency during pregnancy; and rupture of or stretching of the ovarian cortex by the corpus luteum pregnancy. Pain with a threatened miscarriage is due to cramping associated with uterine contractions and cervical dilation. In ectopic pregnancies, the pain can be secondary to tubal distention or hemoperitoneum secondary to rupture of the ectopic. It must be remembered that the "classic triad" of diagnosing ectopic pregnancies (e.g., the combination of amenorrhea, pelvic pain, and pelvic mass) is very nonspecific for an ectopic gestation. Combining the sensitivity of quantitative beta hCG pregnancy testing and transvaginal ultrasonography allows easier and earlier diagnosis of these various pregnancy entities. Frequently, ectopic pregnancies can be diagnosed prior to rupture, thereby allowing medical or minimally invasive surgical treatment and decreasing the risk of major surgery and blood transfusions, as well as better preserving a woman's reproductive potential.

Ovarian Cysts

Ovarian cysts frequently are cited as the cause of the pain when felt on pelvic exam or seen on pelvic ultrasound in the adolescent with pelvic pain. However, the normal function and physiology of the ovary must be remembered, as well as the fact that most ovarian cysts do not cause pain.

Gonadotropins stimulate ovarian follicles through an intricate hormonal process. During the follicular phase, a cohort of follicles are recruited. These follicles mature from primordial follicles to preantral and antral follicles; ultimately, one follicle becomes a preovulatory follicle. The average size of the preovulatory follicle is 2 cm. After ovulation, a corpus luteum is produced from the residual cellular components of the ovulatory follicle. In anovulatory patients, the residual cellular components become a theca luteum. These follicular, corpus luteum, and theca luteum cysts are a product of normal ovarian physiology and hence are labeled physiologic cysts. Functional ovarian cysts are 3-cm or larger fluid-filled ovarian structures that are not neoplastic but the result of gonadatropin stimulation of the ovary. These also can be follicular, corpus luteum, or theca luteum. Physiologic and functional cysts occur in ovulatory and anovulatory cycles and in patients with polycystic ovarian syndrome due to the interplay between gonadatropins, local hormone influence, and cellular receptors. The hormonal mechanisms in these clinical situations differ, due to differences in the positive and negative feedback systems and the secretory patterns of gonadatropins.

Many ovarian cysts, even large ones, do not cause pelvic pain. Theoretically though, there are various mechanisms by which ovarian cysts may cause pain. Rupture of a cyst with spillage of the contents into the peritoneal cavity may cause irritation. When this occurs from the ovulatory follicle, it is called *Mittelschmerz*. This pain from ruptured cysts is typically acute in nature and generally does not persist beyond 24 to 48 hours. If pelvic pain is chronic in nature, it is most likely not secondary to cyst rupture. Pain with ovarian cysts could also theoretically be due to pulling on the adnexal structures. However, in patients with large polycystic ovaries or with ovarian tumors, pelvic pain is rarely a complaint. It is possible that pain associated with cysts could be due to adnexal torsion and de-torsion. The twisting of the blood supply, which can result in intermittent pain, can be associated with ovarian cysts and with other adnexal structures, especially paraovarian cysts. When cysts grow rapidly and thereby stretch the cortex, it is theorized that pain can occur. This can be seen especially in patients undergoing ovulation induction.

Once an ovarian cyst is diagnosed, the method of recommended treatment generally depends on the size of the cyst. The rule of thumb is that cystic masses 7 cm or less in size should be managed conservatively. This recommendation is largely based on a classic study done by Spanous. In this study, cystic masses between the size of 4 and 10 cm in 286 women between the ages of 16 and 48 were treated with a 6-week course of combined estrogens and progesterones. At the completion of 6 weeks, 28% of the masses remained. At the time of surgical exploration, none of these masses were functional ovarian cysts. This treatment produced the following resolution rates: cysts between 4 and 6 cm, 84%; between 6 and 8 cm, 56%; and between 8 and 10 cm, 39%. The estrogen/progesterone therapy suppressed gonadatropin stimulation such that all functional cysts resolved. Further randomized studies, however, have shown that estrogen/progesterone therapy does not hasten the resolution of functional cysts when compared with control groups receiving no therapy. In the female with a cystic mass of 7 cm or less, observation for a 6-week period followed by re-examination will confirm resolution of most cystic masses. In patients without resolution, surgical exploration should then be performed.

Oral contraceptives frequently are used to decrease the risk of ovarian cysts. Studies based on the older, high-dose formulations of oral contraceptives (i.e., ≥50 µg of ethinyl estradiol) demonstrated that oral contraceptives substantially decreased the risk of functional ovarian cysts. Data based on the low-dose formulations widely used today do not support this substantial decrease, as FSH suppression is much less with the low-dose pills than with the high-dose pills. Because patients on progesterone-only pills have a higher incidence of functional cyst formation than women on no exogenous hormones, these are not recommended for suppression of ovarian cysts. The cysts seen in women on progesterone-only contraceptives tend to resolve spontaneously.

Pelvic Inflammatory Disease

Pelvic inflammatory disease (PID) can either be acute or chronic in nature. Diagnosis of PID requires the presence of lower abdominal tenderness, cervical motion tenderness, and adnexal tenderness on exam. In addition, at least one of the following should be present: temperature greater than 38°C, elevated white blood cell count, elevated erythrocyte sedimentation rate, evidence of gonorrhea or chlamydia in the endocervix, inflammatory mass on bimanual pelvic examination, or more than five white blood cells per oil immersion field on gram stain of the endocervical discharge. One should rule out pregnancy although PID is possible very early in pregnancy before the endometrial cavity becomes obliterated with the gestation.

In treating PID, the CDC guidelines should be followed. If one is unsure whether to treat an adolescent with suspected PID as an inpatient or an outpatient, it is better to err on the side of inpatient treatment because of the risks of infertility secondary to tubal damage. Likewise, over-treating soft cases with outpatient therapy also makes sense. In patients treated as outpatients, re-evaluation in 24 to 48 hours is ideal.

It must be remembered that clinical symptoms of PID overlap markedly with the symptoms of other conditions. In patients who have repeatedly been diagnosed with PID, yet have been culture negative, laparoscopy is helpful in establishing the correct diagnosis.

Prevention of infertility is an important objective in treating adolescents with PID. The prevention of infertility is dependent on the time interval between onset of symptoms and treatment. The risk of infertility with PID increases with each episode, being 12% after the first episode, 24% after the second episode, and 48% after the third episode.

Pelvic Adhesions

The role of pelvic adhesions in pelvic pain remains controversial. Some patients with massive adhesions (i.e., a "frozen pelvis") have no pain, whereas some patients with only minimal adhesive disease claim to have intense pain. Many clinicians doubt that adhesions alone cause pain due to the lack of innervation of adhesions. However, adhesions that surround the ovaries or adhesions that involve the bowel may be the type that cause pain.

In young patients, the majority of pelvic adhesions are secondary to pelvic inflammatory disease or appendicitis. While pelvic adhesions may be suspected of causing pelvic pain based upon history and physical exam, adhesions are diagnosed at the time of laparoscopy or laparotomy. Adhesiolysis at the time of surgery is usually performed despite the lack of concrete support in the literature that this is useful. It certainly behooves the clinician to promptly treat both appendicitis and pelvic inflammatory disease because of the long-term sequelae of pelvic adhesions.

Adnexal Torsion

Torsion of the fallopian tube and/or ovary or paraovarian structures is another cause of pelvic pain. The typical presentation is acute onset of unilateral abdominal pain, more frequently on the right side due to the anatomic suspension of the tube and ovary. The pain may be colicky, and there may be a history of similar pain in the past. Nausea and vomiting are associated with the onset of pain in about one fourth of patients. The clinical presentation often is similar to that of appendicitis especially since the right adnexa is more commonly involved. The following characteristics distinguish adnexal torsion and appendicitis:

- With adenexal torsion, the onset of pain is acute, whereas with appendicitis pain tends to be more gradual and periumbilical in onset, then migrating and becoming more acute in the right lower quadrant.
- If nausea is present, it occurs at the onset of pain with ovarian torsion but after the onset of pain with appendicitis.
- Pelvic mass is more commonly felt with ovarian torsion than with appendicitis. Normal ovaries, fallopian tubes, and paraovarian cysts can be involved in torsion.
- On ultrasound, the appendix usually is visible with appendicitis, whereas it is not visible with ovarian tension. If ovarian torsion is associated with a mass, the mass frequently is seen on ultrasound.

The treatment approach to torsion is surgical. Currently, laparoscopy frequently is performed with either removal of the torsed structure or, if it is viable, detorsion of the structure with observation for reestablishment of adequate blood supply. When torsion is due to excessive mobility, oophoropexy (shortening of the supporting ligaments) is recommended to prevent recurrence. If the torsed structure is clearly necrosed and not viable, surgical removal is the recommended treatment.

Dysmenorrhea

The literal meaning of dysmenorrhea is "difficult menstrual flow." Primary dysmenorrhea is painful menstruation in the absence of gross pathology of the pelvic organs. Secondary dysmenorrhea denotes painful menstruation in the presence of underlying pathologic conditions of the pelvic organs (e.g., endometriosis, salpingitis, and congenital anomalies of the mullerian system).

Prostaglandins are the primary cause of the symptoms of dysmenorrhea. It has been shown that menstrual flow of women with dysmenorrhea has a higher prostaglandin level than menstrual flow of women with painless menses. Likewise, the prostaglandin level in menstrual flow and the severity of dysmenorrhea have been correlated. Prostaglandins cause pain by increasing the sensitivity to pain in the nerve terminals, decreasing the blood flow to the uterus, which leads to "uterine angina," and stimulating uterine contractions.

It is of utmost importance to differentiate primary dysmenorrhea from secondary dysmenorrhea. Primary dysmenorrhea has characteristic features that may be obtained in the history. Primary dysmenorrhea is seen after the establishment of ovulatory cycles. Secretory endometrium is the main site of prostaglandin production, which only occurs in ovulatory cycles. It is therefore usually months or years after menarche before dysmenorrhea becomes problematic. Most commonly, primary dysmenorrhea begins 6 to 12 months after menarche. The onset of symptoms may date back to menarche or shortly thereafter. If dysmenorrhea presents later in life, it is usually secondary with an underlying organic cause. The pain with primary dysmenorrhea typically begins several hours before the onset of menses or with the onset of menses. Dysmenorrhea that starts several days before the onset of menses is more commonly secondary dysmenorrhea. The pain is typically described as crampy, spasmodic or labor like, and localized over the lower abdomen and suprapubic region. It maybe described as anything from a dull ache to a sharp stabbing feeling. The pain may radiate to the low back or inner thighs. There may be other symptoms such as diarrhea, headaches, or gastrointestinal distress. Frequently the severity of the pain will have an impact on the adolescent's school work and social activities.

In primary dysmenorrhea, the pelvic examination is essentially normal. The rectal examination is an integral part of the evaluation, as abnormalities of the mullerian system are sometimes only detected with this examination.

The causes of secondary dysmenorrhea include endometriosis, PID, mullerian malformations, ovarian cysts, pelvic adhesions, cervical stenosis, and, although not commonly seen in adolescents, uterine myomas and adenomyosis. With secondary dysmenorrhea, the pelvic examination may reveal a number of signs including adnexal tenderness, ovarian cysts, or abnormalities of the muellerian system. Definitive diagnosis can almost always be established with diagnostic laparoscopy, which frequently will also offer treatment.

Current medical therapy for dysmenorrhea includes antiprostaglandins and oral contraceptives. Antiprostaglandins (prostaglandin synthethase inhibitors) have had a profound impact on the treatment of dysmenorrhea, especially primary dysmenorrhea. They act by inhibiting the production of prostaglandins, providing analgesia, and reducing the edema and erythema associated with inflammation. It is important to use appropriate dose and dosing schedule for maximum effectiveness. The overall effectiveness of prostaglandins in relieving dysmenorrhea is in the 70% range. Oral contraceptives are also very effective in relieving dysmenorrhea. The main mechanism is through suppression of ovulation, thereby preventing formation of the secretory endometrium—the main site of prostaglandin production. Oral contraceptives should be considered in the adolescent with pain unresponsive to prostaglandins and especially in the sexually active teenager. If the patient does not respond to antiprostaglandins and oral contraceptives after a minimum treatment period of 3 months, laparoscopy should be performed. This allows evaluation for an underlying organic cause such as endometriosis as well as therapeutic intervention.

SUMMARY

Acute and chronic pelvic pain in the adolescent patient accounts for a significant number of physician visits. Because an underlying pathologic condition is present in most cases, the adolescent presenting with pelvic pain needs to be taken seriously. Laparoscopy is an important adjunct in the evaluation and treatment of pelvic pain. Adequate diagnosis and early therapy are essential in order to improve the quality of life and to preserve the reproductive prognosis in these young females.

SUGGESTED READINGS

ACOG TECH Bulletin; Chronic Pelvic Pain. ACOG Technical Bulletin 129: June 1989.

Chattan DL; Ward AB: Endometriosis in Adolescents. J. Reprod. Med 27: 156, 1982.

Davis G. Clinical characteristics of adolescent endometriosis. J Adol Health 1993; 14:362–368.

Fried-Oginski W. Pelvic inflammatory disease in adolescents. Adol Ped Gynecology (1992) 5:243–247.

Gidwani GP: Laparoscopy for diagnosis of chronic pelvic pain. Transitions 1981: December. Goldstein DP, DeCholnoky C, Emans SJ, et al. Laparoscopy in the diagnosis and management of pelvic pain in adolescents. J Reprod Med 1980; 24:251.

Goldstein DP, Pinsonneault O: Pelvic Pain in the Pediatric and Adolescent Patient; Clinical Practice of Gynecology:3, 137/145, 1989.

Howard FM. The role of laparoscopy in chronic pelvic pain: Promise and Pitfalls. Obstet and Gynecol Survey 48: 6, 1993.

Merritt D: Torsion of the uterine adnexae: a review. Adolesc Pediatr Gynecol (1991) 4:3–13.

Smith RP: The dynamics of nonsteroidal anti-inflammatory therapy for primary dysmenorrhea. Obstet Gynecol 70:785, 1987.

Spanos WJ: Preoperative hormonal therapy of cystic adnexal masses AM J Obstet Gynecol 116:4, p. 551–556, 1973.

Swee: RC: Pelvic inflammatory disease and infertility in women; Infect Dis Clin North Am 1:199–215. 1987.

INDEX

A

Abdominal pain
    and adnexal torsion, 93
    diagnostic testing, 89–90
    differential diagnosis, 88
    and dysmenorrhea, 93–94
    history of patient, 87–89
    and ovarian cysts, 90–92
    and pelvic adhesions, 92
    and pelvic inflammatory disease (PID), 92
    physical examination, 89
    and pregnancy, 90
Abnormal uterine bleeding
    acute episode, treatment, 66, 67
    and cervical lesions, 64
    and coagulation defects, 63
    common cause in adolescent, 64–65
    and endocrine disorders, 63
    history of patient, 64–65
    hormonal therapy, 67
    hospitalization, 66–67
    and human papilloma virus (HPV), 64
    hypomenorrhea, 64
    and infection, 64
    laboratory studies, 65–66
    and malignancy, 64
    and medication use, 63–64
    menometrorrhagia, 64
    menorrhagia, 64
    metorrhagia, 64
    oligomenorrhea, 64
    physical exam, 65
    and polycystic ovarian disease, 64
    polymenorrhea, 64
    and pregnancy, 64
    and systemic disease, 63
    treatment of, 66–67
    and vaginal lesions, 64
Acne, 72
Addison's disease, and abnormal uterine bleeding, 63
Adnexal torsion
    and abdominal pain, 93
    compared to appendicitis, 93
    treatment of, 93
Adolescent development
    areas of, 74
    genital tract development, 20–21
    tasks of, 74
Adolescent patient
    breast exam, 17
    and confidentiality, 16–17
    examination process, 17
    explanation of exam to, 17
    and hidden agendas, 16
    interview with patient, 16–17
    laboratory testing, 17–18
    mother, interview with, 15–16
    positioning of, 17
    post-exam counseling, 18
    rapport with patient, 16
    and sexual abuse, 16
    speculum for, 17
Adolescent sexuality
    in early adolescence, 74